Bladder Augmentation

Edited by

Paddy Dewan PhD MS MD FRCS FRACS
Paediatric Urology Unit, Royal Children's Hospital,
Melbourne, Australia

Michael E Mitchell MD
Division of Urology, Children's Hospital and
Medical Center, University of Washington School of
Medicine, Seattle, USA

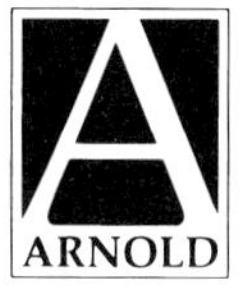

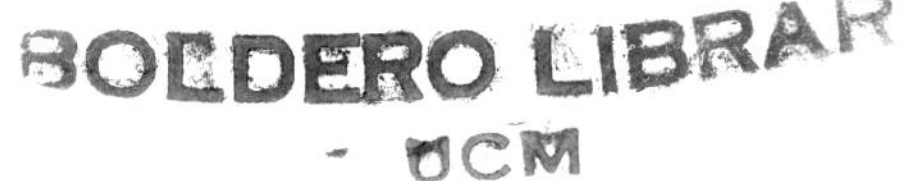

A member of the Hodder Headline Group
LONDON
Co-published in the United States of America by
Oxford University Press Inc., New York

First published in Great Britain in 2000 by
Arnold, a member of the Hodder Headline Group,
338 Euston Road, London NW1 3BH

http://www.arnoldpublishers.com

Co-published in the United States of America by
Oxford University Press Inc.,
198 Madison Avenue, New York, NY10016
Oxford is a registered trademark of Oxford University Press

British Library Cataloguing in Publication Data
A catalogue record for this book is available from the British Library

Library of Congress Cataloging-in-Publication Data
A catalog record for this book is available from the Library of Congress

ISBN 0 340 75957 7

1 2 3 4 5 6 7 8 9 10

Commissioning Editor: Nick Dunton
Production Editor: Rada Radojicic
Production Controller: Iain McWilliams
Cover Design: Terry Griffiths

Typeset in 10/12 Minion
Composition by Scribe Design, Gillingham, Kent
Colour reproduction Tenon & Polert Colour Scanning Ltd, Hong Kong
Printed and bound in Great Britain by Bath Press, Bath

What do you think about this book? Or any other Arnold title?
Please send your comments to feedback.arnold@hodder.co.uk

Contents

Colour plate section appears between pages 86 and 87

Contributors

Laurence S Baskin MD
Pediatric Urology, UCSF School of Medicine, San Francisco, CA, USA

David A Bloom MD
Division of Pediatric Urology, University of Michigan Medical Center, Ann Arbor, MI, USA

Michael C Carr PhD MD
Division of Urology, Children's Hospital of Philadelphia, University of Pennsylvania, Philadelphia, PA, USA

Patrick Cartwright MD
Urology Department, Children's Medical Center, Salt Lake City, UT, USA

Earl Y Cheng MD
Division of Pediatric Urology, Children's Hospital of Oklahoma, Oklahoma City, OK, USA

Clare E Close MD
Children's Urology Associates, 3201 S. Maryland Pkwy, Suite #406, Las Vegas, NV, USA

Gerald Cunha MD
Pediatric Urology Center, UCSF School of Medicine, San Francisco, CA, USA

Paddy Dewan PhD MS MD FRCS FRACS
Paediatric Urology Unit, Royal Children's Hospital, Melbourne, Australia

Peter Frey MD BSc
Service de Chirurgie Pédiatrique, Centre Hospitalier Universitaire Vaudois, Lausanne, Switzerland

Ricardo González MD
Division of Pediatric Urology, University of Miami, Miami, FL, USA

Richard W Grady MD
Division of Urology, Children's Hospital and Medical Center, University of Washington School of Medicine, Seattle, WA, USA

Roman Jednak MD
Division of Pediatric Urology, Montreal Children's Hospital, Montreal, Canada

William E Kaplan MD
Department of Urology, Northwestern University, Children's Memorial Hospital, Chicago, IL, USA

Bradley P Kropp MD
Division of Pediatric Urology, Children's Hospital of Oklahoma, Oklahoma City, OK, USA

Christian Lorenz MD
Kinderchirurgische Universitätsklinik, Mannheim, Germany

Nicolas Lutz MD
Service de Chirurgie Pédiatrique, Centre Hospitalier Universitaire Vaudois, Lausanne, Switzerland

Gordon A Mclorie MD
Division of Urology, Hospital for Sick Children, Toronto, Canada

Michael E Mitchell MD
Division of Urology, Children's Hospital and Medical Center, University of Washington School of Medicine, Seattle, WA, USA

John M Park MD
Division of Pediatric Urology, University of Michigan Medical Center, Ann Arbor, MI, USA

Joao Luiz Pippi Salle MD PhD
Division of Pediatric Urology, Montreal Children's Hospital, Montreal, Canada

Richard C Rink MD
Division of Pediatric Urology, James Whitcombe Reilly Hospital for Sick Children, Indiana University Medical Center, Indianapolis, IN, USA

Brent Snow MD
Urology Department, Children's Medical Center, Salt Lake City, UT, USA

Thomas S Vates MD
Department of Pediatric Urology, Children's Hospital of Michigan, Detroit, MI, USA

Foreword

Forty years ago I was about to start a year as an exchange fellow in Chicago and was casting about for an idea for a research project, when Richard Turner-Warwick happened to tell me about Shoemaker's claims to be able to grow urothelium over raw ileum from which the mucosa had been scraped off. In those days ureterosigmoidostomy was the standard method of urinary diversion and the wards were full of long-term survivors suffering from the hyperchloraemic acidosis which resulted when urine was absorbed by intestinal mucosa. All over the world research was being carried out to understand and prevent this distressing complication. In Chicago, Gilchrist and Merricks had described an isolated pouch which was said to provide continence and avoid acidosis. To reline the bowel with waterproof urothelium seemed to offer an ideal solution.

In Chicago I was given every facility to attempt to reproduce Shoemaker's work, and in addition was afforded the privilege of following up the patients of Drs Gilchrist and Merricks.

It was then that I learned why every surgeon needs to have a little go at research. Nothing else teaches the lesson that what is printed ain't necessarily so. I learned that it was impossible to scrape the mucosa off the bowel; you had to take the submucosa as well. The idea that urothelium could magically transform underlying connective tissue into detrusor muscle turned out to be an optimistic misinterpretation of the histology; in fact, the muscle fibres arose by regeneration from the stump of the canine bladder. Patients with ileocaecal pouches were seldom continent, often had infection, calculi and hyperchloraemic acidosis, and during my year there the operation seemed to have been given up.

Today, in spite of 30 more years of research, the ideal substitute for the urinary bladder remains tantalisingly out of reach. Practically every tissue (not excluding dura mater) has been used to replace all or part of the bladder; none of them works. Indeed, the difficulties of the problem that faces us have multiplied during a period which has brought new histochemical techniques and the whole new technology of urodynamics. Hitherto unsuspected networks of nerves with their own chemical transmitters have been discovered. There has been considerable experience with electrical stimulation or division of sacral nerve roots. There have been so many reinventions and variations on the pioneer *néovessies* of Gil-Vernet, Couvelaire and Kuss that hardly a university hospital does not have its own pet-named version; sufficient testimony that none of them is perfect. To find the answer will need much more research and many more young surgeons. To them this book will be an invaluable springboard.

It will also appeal to a wider readership of urologists who want to keep up to date; they will marvel at the remarkable effect that dilatation of the urethra is said to have upon the long-term function of the neuropathic detrusor, and of electrical stimulation on its growth; but it is invidious to pick out only one or two plums from a cake which is so rich in them. This book is a goldmine of information; how I wish I had had something like it 40 years ago.

John Blandy CBE, FRCS
London

Preface

> ... there remain many considerable discoveries to be made .... This may encourage us not to despond, if we do not find all enquires attended by discoveries.
>
> Cowper, W. (1699)
> *Philos Tr Roy Soc London*, **258**, 364–9

Cowper penned the above words well before the development of either urinary diversion or bladder augmentation, and he was referring to the urethra, not the bladder. However, 300 years later, the sentiment is relevant to researchers and clinicians involved in the field of bladder augmentation who need to remember that a perfect solution is still not available, and new techniques are rapidly coming on line. Those who are involved in advising parents of children about management of the neurogenic bladder will be aware of the increasing difficulty of giving advice to patients because of the large number of alternative surgical and non-surgical treatments of incontinence. The alternative therapies have been collected in this one volume, to highlight the difficulty of deciding which might be the best treatment for a small high-pressure bladder. We have also indicated the research which is being pursued in attempting to improve the outcome for the continence and renal function of these individuals.

The journey through the options and related research starts with a chapter on the history of bladder augmentation surgery, which was felt important, particularly because it appears that many of the lessons learnt in the laboratory, and from the treatment of patients, are often not taken into account when workers embark on the development of new techniques. We end with the latest developments in tissue regeneration and explore the multiple operative and non-operative approaches between the two end-points. A particular focus has been on producing a urothelial urinary reservoir, while still satisfying the important aims of preserving renal parenchyma and producing continence. Nevertheless, small bowel, large bowel, gastric segment and gut mucosa lined augmentation techniques and results are presented for completeness.

Further research is likely to provide insight into the advantages and disadvantages of the new, the old and the future innovations; careful, open-minded interpretation of clinical and laboratory results will ultimately lead to a range of therapies being combined differently for each neurogenic bladder patient. The bladder management which is most easily applied and least likely to result in failure or complications will become the most used in the future. As yet the panacea for bladder augmentation has not been found. It is hoped that this book will educate some and encourage others to further the research

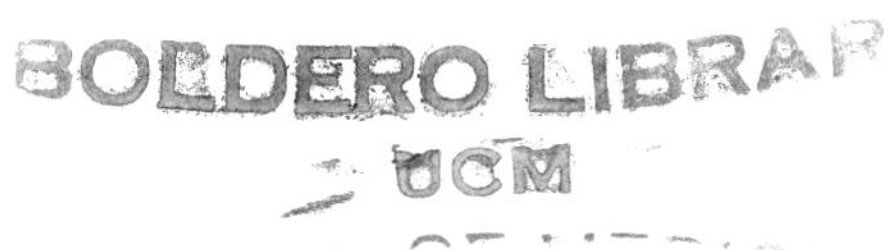

1

The history of bladder augmentation

CHRISTIAN LORENZ

INTRODUCTION

One hundred years ago the first successful attempts to use bowel segments for the augmentation of the human urinary bladder were reported. In 1898, Rutkowski in Krakow and Mikulicz in Breslau operated on older children for bladder exstrophy. Rutkowski performed a one-stage ileocystoplasty;[1] Mikulicz was more cautious, preferring a delayed two-stage operation.[2] It appears that Mikulicz was rightly cautious, given the inconsistent results of several animal studies as well as the poor results of the first attempts to preserve isolated vascularized intestinal segments in humans (mainly for the treatment of gut disorders). In 1889, Tizzoni and Foggi from Bologna reported successful orthotopic replacement of the urinary bladder in dogs; they anastomosed intestinal loops to the bladder neck and performed subsequent bilateral ureteric reimplantation.[3] However, only one out of eight dogs survived the one-stage operation. On the other hand, success with urinary diversion into colon, rectum, or intestinal conduits had already been published by Maydl, Giordano, Mauclaire, Gersuny, Krynski and others cited by Rutkowski.[1] In 1852, Simon reported the first ureterosigmoidostomy in humans.[4]

Thus, the beginning of a century of bladder augmentation appears to have been as controversial as its end. However, with respect to bladder augmentation, statements from early proponents are still valid. Rutkowski wrote in 1899: 'A bowel wall patch, pedicled on the mesentery, meets all these requirements; with it we, therefore, have the ideal material for a cystoplasty;'[1] and Mikulicz, also in 1899, cautioned that 'the value of it [the operative technique] is finally, however, only dependent on the subsequent function of the created bladder.[2] Obviously, as for the initial studies, any subsequent progress in the field of bladder augmentation and replacement will be influenced by continued basic research and the use of animal models.

ROUTINE ENTEROCYSTOPLASTY

Many technical variations, based on the principle of detubularization of an isolated bowel loop, have been advocated and clinically applied since the initial work of Rutkowski, Mikulicz and others.[5] The progress in surgery and the development of operative urology, internal medicine, radiology, obstetrics, and pediatrics have helped further to broaden the clinical indications for enterocystoplasties, which now include bladder wall changes due to inflammation (tuberculosis, interstitial cystitis), neoplasms, the treatment of congenital anomalies (bladder exstrophy, COPUM bladder), and neurogenic bladder associated with myelodysplasia. The use of various bowel segments, such as ileum,[6–9] ileocecum,[10–12] cecum,[5,13,14] and sigmoid colon,[15–21] produced comparable functional results for the bladder.[8,20,22–8] The operative principles of incorporation of intestinal segments into the lower urinary tract were refined to meet the clinical demands for augmentation, substitution, or replacement bladder.[29] Therefore, the bowel segments are sutured to the bladder in a variety of ways, including after longitudinal[6,30,31] or crossed bladder incision,[32] or after folding and resuturing of the bowel patch into spherical cup-like structures;[6,33] whereas, for bladder replacement, reshaping of bowel segments with or without antireflux measures is preferred.[34–6] The volume of the augmented bladder is predictable using geometrical and physical formulae.[37,38] In the recent past, additional treatment modalities, such as anticholinergic drugs, clean intermittent catheterization,[39] creation of catheterizable channels,[40–2] and advanced management of bladder outlet resistance by endoscopic augmentation techniques[43–5] or the use of artificial urinary sphincter systems,[46–9] have altered the indications for, and improved the outcome of, bladder augmentation. In pediatric patients, a trend toward undiversion, a term coined by Hendren in 1973,[50] was also based on the expectation that enterocystoplasty gives a better renal prognosis than upper urinary tract diversion.[51–53]

Because the literature on the urodynamic function of various types of enterocystoplasties is extensive and heterogeneous, preference for a particular technique cannot be scientifically decided. However, hard data on risks and complications of enterocystoplasty have been collected over the years and should be considered whenever an enterocystoplasty is contemplated. These include excessive mucous production, recurrent urinary tract infection, reflux or obstruction at the vesicoureteric junction, metabolic changes (acidosis, ammonemia), and electrolyte shifts (hyperchloremia, hypercalcuria).[28,29,54–61] More recently, spontaneous bladder perforation, hematological changes, and growth retardation have been recognized,[62–5] along with the risk of malignancy, bone demineralization, chronic vitamin deficiency, urinary stone formation, fibrosis, and bone formation within the intestinal segments.[66–74] The reported incidence of complications related to the use of intestinal segments varies widely, dependent on age, basic disease, type of enteroplasty, and renal function.

GASTROCYSTOPLASTY

The technique of isolation of a vascularized segment from stomach was established in the nineteenth century by the German physiologist Heidenhain (1834–97), who used his model to study gastric secretion. However, it was the recognition of the nonabsorbing quality of the gastric segment that inspired Sinaiko in 1953 to use the Heidenhain pouch for urinary diversion in dogs, and subsequently in humans.[75,76] Metabolic and infection problems, observed with other types of urinary diversion such as ureterosigmoidostomy[77–9] or intestinal conduits,[80] were thought potentially to be reduced by the use of the stomach. Consistent with this is the fact that Sinaiko focused on the metabolic consequences, secretory behavior, and regulation of the gastric pouch rather than on its storage ability, which he obviously never questioned. To take advantage of the preventative effect of acid urine on urinary calculus disease, Martin *et al.* autografted gastric mucosa into the bladder.[81] In 1962, Martin *et al.* were the first to report a series of gastrocystoplasties in dogs by adapting the gastric pedicle to allow the segment to reach the orthotopic bladder. The part of the stomach used, the method of fashioning both the segment and its blood supply, and the secretory consequences have since been further studied.[82–5] Karow and Thompson in 1969 carried out a study in dogs, adding a previously created gastric pouch to a pouch sigmoidostomy in order to influence both the inflammatory and metabolic side-effects of ureterosigmoidostomy.[86] Further work on the potentially favorable effect of gastric acid secretion on the net chloride excretion in patients with hyperchloremic acidosis demonstrated advantages from using stomach instead of colon in the case of chronic renal failure.[87] Adams and coworkers therefore advocated the use of gastrocystoplasty in patients with compromised renal function and metabolic acidosis.[88] Extensive work has looked at both the potential and the real risks of gastrocystoplasty, including: (a) serum gastrin changes and their relationship to the specific portion of the stomach and the effect of distension; (b) the effect of acid output on metabolism and the remaining bladder; (c) mucus production; (d) stone formation; and (e) the development of bladder ulceration.[64,81,85,87,89–93]

To date, marked symptoms due to acid in the bladder and urethra are the most important complication in gastrocystoplasty patients.[94–6] Many of those with symptoms need to have both systemic acid-blocking medication (H2–receptor antagonists, proton pump inhibitors) and bladder irrigations with buffer solutions to neutralize urine pH. Since long-term follow-up is still lacking, only animal studies in rats suggest the risk of metaplasia in both the adjacent urothelium and the incorporated segment of gastric mucosa,[64] warranting lifelong follow-up for these patients. Nevertheless, for selected patients, and children in particular, there is increasing evidence that the majority of reported gastrocystoplasties improved the urodynamic bladder function.[97–104] This success in rather difficult clinical situations, together with a reduced overall risk, has to be taken into account when considering the options for bladder enlargement. Further information on the use and success of gastrocystoplasty is given in Chapter 6.

SEROMUSCULAR CYSTOPLASTY

In 1955, Shoemaker was awarded first prize by the American Urological Association for an essay on bladder augmentation experiments in dogs using seromuscular intestinal segments.[105] His group advocated removal of the mucosal lining, leaving a raw muscular and serosal vascularized graft; the detubularized segment was used as both reversed and nonreversed segments for bladder reconstruction,[106,107] on which they identified growth and differentiation of urothelium within 2–3 weeks. These findings were in line with those of Neuhof,[108] who demonstrated urothelial ingrowth over fascial grafts used to repair surgical defects in the bladder wall of experimental animals. Furthermore, the two-layered muscular architecture of the intestine interlaced into a plexiform network, indistinguishable from normal detrusor muscle. Campbell was the first to perform a de-epithelialized intestinocystoplasty in a patient.[109] Later, Martin performed further animal experiments using a mucosa-free ileal loop subtotal bladder substitution.[110] He reported a slower regrowth of the transitional epithelium (4 to 5 weeks) than indicated by Shoemaker's group, but confirmed changes in the muscle architecture of the ileal patch. Subsequent animal studies, using ileum and colon, with either the serosal or denuded external wall covering the inner surface of the bladder, have shown mixed results.[111–16] The ingrowth of urothelium does occur within 3 to 6 weeks in most studies, depending on the extent of the remaining bladder and the species used. However, the slow ingrowth allows inflammation and fibrosis of the muscle patch, resulting in shrinkage. Also, calculus formation and regeneration of the bowel mucosa occur. The mucosa is difficult to remove from the small and large bowel, increasing the chances of regrowth of the gastrointestinal epithelum. However, mechanical trauma during complete denudation of the muscle may be responsible for the fibrotic changes seen.[117,118] Therefore, more gentle techniques of mucosa removal have been described without a definitive solution for application in humans so far being achieved.[119,120] Since removal of mucosa from gastric segments appeared easier, this was used in a comparative animal study serving as a control for a combined augmentation procedure.[121,122] However, fibrosis and shrinkage were again observed if the urothelial lining was achieved by urothelial ingrowth. This may explain why Blandy's optimistic outlook on the clinical use of seromuscular intestinal segments, which he considered as 'dry, safe and acceptable,'[111] has not resulted because of the fibrosis. Pompino *et al.*[123] cited Russian authors who used seromuscular grafts in children with a neurogenic bladder. Reinnervationplasty, vesicopexy, and autocystoduplication were the names used to describe their attempts to attach a seromuscular ileal patch to the back of the bladder after removal of its serosa. Even though a number of children were reported to be treated successfully by these workers, Pompino *et al.* could not confirm the optimistic results obtained in Russia. All these latter studies were mainly aimed at reinnervation of the bladder.

UROTHELIAL-LINED BLADDER AUGMENTATION

Huggins in 1931 described the removal of a patch of detrusor muscle, preserving the continuity of the urothelial lining, and the suturing of fascia into the muscle defect.[124] This prevented bone formation seen by Neuhof[108] and others when the fascial graft came into direct contact with urine. Huggins also performed transplantation of urothelial patches into other abdominal sites focusing on the mechanisms of bone formation. Subsequently, Martin was the first to report transplantation of a bladder mucosa strip which he had removed from the resected bladder to attach to the inner surface of a demucosalized ileal segment in dogs:[110] the urothelium survived and appeared to hasten the uroepithelialization of the ileal bladder. Reviewing the literature and adding his own experimental data, Blandy in 1964 emphasized the unique property of urothelium: it is almost waterproof and allows only minimal movement of water and ions, making it perfect for lining a urinary reservoir.[111] This recognition may have helped foster further attempts to find ways to perform a urothelial-lined bladder augmentation. Current attempts reflecting the importance of an intact urothelial lining are aimed at preservation of intact urothelium instead of regeneration.

Mau reported in 1980 on the creation of a neuropathic bladder in pigs and subsequent surgical removal of two-thirds of the spastic and trabeculated bladder muscle, leaving the urothelial layer intact. A detubularized seromuscular ileal segment was then sewn over the urothelium, producing a urothelial-lined ileal graft. Histopathological investigation showed an intact transitional epithelium attached to the muscular layer of the ileal patch in most specimens, with only mild inflammation between the two layers. The results were considered unfavorable because the muscle did not become reinnervated.[125] Mau, however, demonstrated encouraging results for the capacity and compliance of the bladder. This was before clean intermittent catheterization became available as a way of emptying these nonfunctioning bladder reservoirs.

Autoaugmentation,[126] detrusorectomy,[127,128] autocystoplasty,[129] vesicomyotomy,[130] detrusormyotomy, and partial detrusor excision[131] are terms for a single principle: an incision in the bladder muscle, similar to the routine clam cystoplasty, which does not breach the bladder mucosa, which is allowed to bulge through the muscle incision as a wide-mouthed diverticulum. Cartwright and Snow were the first to report their results in dogs[126] and then in a series of patients.[132] Their microscopic investigations in dogs 4 to 6 weeks after operation showed scarring over the bladder dome where the detrusor had been resected, but the urothelial layer, lamina propria, and network of small vessels were intact, although surrounded by a thin layer of collagen and a layer of hypercellular fibrous tissue. Shrinking of the urothelial bulge with time has meant that the long-term results of this technique have not been favorable. Small, trabeculated bladders respond less well to autoaugmentation and there appears to be a risk of vesicoureteric reflux and bladder perforation. Nevertheless, several groups reported good results with this technique in a number of children[128,130] and adults,[133,134] even when combined with other surgical steps such as the creation of a Mitrofanoff stoma or ureteric reimplants.[134,135] Furthermore, this is the only bladder augmentation technique to date allowing minimal invasive application.[136]

To reduce the risk of adverse changes to the autoaugmented bladder in the long term, Dewan *et al.* introduced a supplementary backing of the urothelium by seromuscular segments from stomach or colon, first in a sheep model,[117,137] the long-term results of which justified clinical use.[138,139] At the same time, this extension of the original autoaugmentation was used increasingly, mainly in pediatric patients.[140–3] However, the success of this combined procedure seems to depend on the feasibility of autoaugmentation initially. Thus, careful patient selection is required because autoaugmentation and derived techniques are not appropriate for severely shrunken bladders.

Other techniques utilizing urothelial-lined tissues include diverticulocystoplasty[144] and ureterocystoplasty,[53,145–152] which preserve structures that would often previously have been resected. Their integration into the bladder, although only occasionally possible, can postpone or eliminate the need for more extensive bladder augmentation. Ureterocystoplasty is further described in Chapter 8.

Having summarized studies of urothelial-lined seromuscular segment bladder augmentation, efforts to regenerate the bladder are worth mentioning. Spontaneous regeneration of the bladder after subtotal resection was observed in animals in the late nineteenth century by Tizzoni and Foggi[3] and Schwarz.[153] Perlmann had similar findings in dogs after complete bladder resection.[154] However, this strategy of avoiding the incorporation of gut or urinary diversion after near-total bladder loss had only been reported in humans. In 1963, Tucci and Haralambidis summarized 28 cases recorded up to that date in the literature.[155] The outcome was poor for the required time for bladder reconfiguration, the extent of extravasation, subsequent infection, and the capacity and compliance of the neobladder. Therefore, numerous studies were instigated to use biological or synthetic materials as prostheses for subsequent bladder regeneration. Neuhof in 1917[156] and Huggins in 1932[124] replaced the bladder wall with fascia; Kelami renewed attempts to replace parts of the bladder wall by using lyophilized human dura. He published a series of 37 patients and noted the adoption of the technique by other groups: he confirmed complete absorption of the dura, but urothelial covering of the bladder lumen.[157] Others have similarly employed peritoneum,[158] myoperitoneum,[159,160] omentum,[161] and bovine pericardium;[162,163] again, complete epithelialization could be confirmed, but none of these artificial materials has led to a breakthrough.[164,165] Stanley *et al.* reported the incorporation of a thin-walled silastic cup lined with Dacron velour in sheep and dogs,[166] and Fishman *et al.* documented the use of fresh placental membranes as a scaffold for bladder enlargement in dogs.[167] Swinney stated that although artificial materials may be used to replace the bladder, they do not really become incorporated, thus acting only as scaffold for urothelium and fibrous tissue; satisfactory function in such cases is achieved by the adaptation of the remaining tissues and not by regeneration of muscle.[168]

TISSUE ENGINEERING TECHNIQUES

Recent understanding of the role and composition of extracellular tissue matrix has led to cell and tissue culture and subsequent replacement *in vivo*. Bladder regeneration technology has stemmed from the preparation of acellular tissue matrix from rat stomach or bladder and its syngeneic use by Sutherland *et al.*,[169] the isolation of porcine small intestinal submucosa by Badylak *et al.*,[170] and its subsequent use for bladder augmentation in rats and dogs by Kropp *et al.*,[171–3] Probst *et al* have isolated bladder acellular matrix graft from rat bladder and used it to replace the bladder dome in rats.[174] All groups documented not only regeneration of bladder urothelium and smooth muscle but also vascular and neural regeneration.

Cell culture techniques, developed from Rheinwald and Green's work on human keratinocytes,[174] have been adopted for urothelial cell culture in both human and several animal models.[176–82] The introduction of matrices for growth *in vivo*, such as collagen membrane or gel,[183,184] biodegradable meshes,[185,186] or films of lactidcapro-lactoncopolymer,[186] made the application to *in vivo* studies possible. Transplantation of cultured urothelium onto seromuscular segments and immediate bladder incorporation failed,[187] or did not produce satisfactory[186] survival and proliferation of the cells *in vivo*. However, a recent study confirmed the development of a differentiated urothelial lining on seromuscular segments of stomach and colon in the absence of urothelium-bearing structures.[188] More complex tissue engineering, such as the experimental incorporation of cultured bladder urothelial and muscle cells on a biodegradable carrier by Atala *et al.*,[185] has not yet been used in humans. Like Atala's group, which is 'aggressively pursuing further work in both the molecular and in vivo realms in order to accomplish the goal of human applicability,'[189] there is ongoing research in this field worldwide, including the techniques presented and discussed in Chapter 15.

REFERENCES

1. Rutkowski, M. (1899) Zur Methode der Harnblasenplastik. *Zentralblatt fur Chirurgie,* **16**, 473–8.
2. Mikulicz, J. (1899) Zur Operation der angeborenen Blasenspalte. *Zentralblatt fur Chirurgie,* **26,** 641–3.
3. Tizzoni, G. and Foggi, A. (1888) Die Wiederherstellung der Harnblase. Experimentelle Untersuchungen. *Zentralblatt fur Chirurgie,* **15**, 921–4.
4. Simon, J. (1852) Ectopia vesicae – absence of the anterior walls of the bladder and pubic abdominal parieties – operation for directing the orifices of the ureters into the rectum, temporary success, subsequent death, autopsy. *Lancet,* **2**, 256–68.
5. Couvelaire, R. (1950) La 'petite vessie' des tuberculeaux genito-urinaires. Essai de classification place et variantes des cysto-intestino-plasties. *Journal d'Urologie,* **56**, 641.
6. Tasker, J.H. (1953) Ileo-cystoplasty: a new technique. An experimental study with report of a case. *British Journal of Urology,* **25**, 349–57.
7. Cibert, J. and Durand, L. (1956) The treatment of certain cases of neurogenic bladder by substitute ileocystoplasty. *British Journal of Urology,* **28**, 301–3.
8. Pike, J.G., Berardinucci, G., Hamburger, B. *et al.* (1991) The surgical management of urinary incontinence in myelodysplastic children. *Journal of Pediatric Surgery*, **26**, 466–71.
9. Goodwin, W.E., Turner, R.D. and Winter, C.C. (1958) Results of ileocystoplasty. *Journal of Urology,* **80**, 461–6.
10. Gilchrist, R.K., Merricks, J.W., Hamlin, H.H. *et al.* (1950) Construction of a substitute bladder and urethra. *Surgery, Gynecology & Obstetrics,* **90**, 752–7.
11. Merricks, J.W. and Gilchrist, R.K. (1954) The ileocecal segment as a substitute bladder; a review of 18 cases. *Journal of Urology*, **71**, 591–8.
12. Gil-Vernet, J.M. (1965) The ileocolic segment in urologic surgery. *Journal of Urology,* **94**, 418–26.
13. Zinman, L. and Libertino, J.A. (1980) Technique of augmentation cecocystoplasty. *Surgery Clinics of North America*, **60**, 703–10.
14. Benchekroun, A. (1977) Continent caecal bladder. *European Urology*, **3**, 248–50.
15. Winter, C.C. and Goodwin, W.E. (1958) Results of sigmoidocystoplasty. *Journal of Urology,* **80**, 467–74.
16. Kuess, R. (1959) Colo-cystoplasty rather than ileo-cystoplasty. *Journal of Urology,* **82**, 587–9.
17. Gregoir, W. (1961) Special indications for colocystoplasty and total colic substitute bladder. *International Urology,* **11**, 328–41.
18. Heeg, M.M., Chappell, S.M. and Paries, W.J. (1968) The use of intact colon to expand bladder capacity. *Journal of Urology,* **99**, 436–8.
19. Kuess, R. (1958) La colo-cystoplastie. A propos de 15 cas. *Journal d'Urologie et Nephrologie*, **64**, 201–7.
20. Morales, P.A., Ong, G., Askari, S. *et al.* (1958) Sigmoidocystoplasty for the contracted bladder. *Journal of Urology,* **80,** 455–60.
21. Beseghi, U., Casolari, E., Del Rossi, C. *et al.* (1994) Enterocystoplasty with a sigmoid patch in children with neurogenic bladder dysfunction. *Pediatric Surgery International*, **9**, 82–5.
22. Dounis, A. and Gow, J.G. (1979) Bladder augmentation – a long-term review. *British Journal of Urology*, **51**, 264–8.
23. Sethia, K.K., Webb, R.J. and Neal, D.E. (1991) Urodynamic study of ileocystoplasty in the treatment of idiopathic detrusor instability. *British Journal of Urology*, **67,** 286–90.
24. Tammela, T.L.J., Lindell, O.I., Viitanen, J.K. *et al.* (1991) Functional and urodynamic characteristics of bladder substitution with detubularised right colonic segment. *British Journal of Urology,* **67**, 298–302.
25. Charghi, A., Charbonneau, J. and Gauthier, G-E. (1967) Colocystoplasty for bladder enlargement and bladder substitution: a study of late results in 31 cases. *Journal of Urology,* **97**, 849–56.
26. Goldwasser, B., Barrett, D.M., Webster, G.D. *et al.* (1987) Cystometric properties of ileum and right colon after bladder augmentation, substitution or replacement. *Journal of Urology,* **138**, 1007–8.

27. Urban, D.A., Kerbl, K., Clayman, R.V. *et al.* (1994) Endo-ureteroplasty with a free urothelial graft. *Journal of Urology,* **152**, 910–15.
28. Hasan, S.T., Marshall, C., Robson, W.A. *et al.* (1995) Clinical outcome and quality of life following enterocystoplasty for idiopathic detrusor instability and neurogenic bladder dysfunction. *British Journal of Urology,* **76**, 551–7.
29. Goldwasser, B. and Webster, G.D. (1986) Augmentation and substitution enterocystoplasty. *Journal of Urology,* **135**, 215–24.
30. Bramble, F.J. (1982) The treatment of adult enuresis and urge incontinence by enterocystoplasty. *British Journal of Urology,* **54**, 693–6.
31. Mundy, A.R. and Stephenson, T.P. (1985) Clam ileocystoplasty for the treatment of refractory urge incontinence. *British Journal of Urology,* **57**, 641–6.
32. Keating, M.A., Ludlow, J.K. and Rich, M.A. (1996) Enterocystoplasty: the star modification. *Journal of Urology,* **155,** 1723–5.
33. Goodwin, W.E., Winter, C.C. and Baker, W.F. (1959) 'Cup-patch' technique of ileocystoplasty for bladder enlargement or partial substitution. *Surgery, Gynecology and Obstetrics,* **108**, 240–4.
34. Robertson, G.N. and King, L. (1986) Bladder substitution in children. *Urology Clinics of North America,* **13**, 333–6.
35. Muller, S.C., Riedmiller, H., Throff, J. *et al.* (1991) Bladder augmentation and continent urinary diversion with use of the appendix, in Marshall, F.F. (ed). *Operative Urology.* Philadelphia, Saunders: 157–8.
36. Rogers, E. and Scardino, P.T. (1995) A simple ileal substitute bladder after radical cystectomy: experience with a modification of the studer pouch. *Journal of Urology,* **153**, 1432–8.
37. Hinman, F. (1988) Selection of intestinal segments for blader substitution: physical and physiological characteristics. *Journal of Urology,* **139**, 519–23.
38. Koff, S.A. (1988) Guidelines to determine the size and shape of intestinal segments used for reconstruction. *Journal of Urology,* **140**, 1150–1.
39. Lapides, J., Diokno, A.C., Lowe, B.S. *et al.* (1974) Followup on unsterile intermittent self-catheterisation. *Journal of Urology,* **111**, 184–7.
40. Verhoogen, J. (1908) Neostomic uretero-cecale formation d'une nouvelle pouche vesicale et d'un nouvel uretre. *Association Française d'Urologie,* **12**, 549–52.
41. Mitrofanoff, P. (1980) Cystostomie continente trans-appendiculaire dans le traitement des vessies neurologiques. *Chirurgie Pediatrique,* **21,** 297–305.
42. Woodhouse, C.R.J. and Macneily, A.E. (1994) The Mitrofanoff principle: expanding upon a versatile technique. *British Journal of Urology,* **74**, 447–53.
43. Vorstman, B., Lockhart, J., Kaufman, M.R. *et al.* (1985) Polytetrafluoroethylene injection for urinary incontinence in children. *Journal of Urology,* **133**, 248–50.
44. Politano, V.A., Small, M.P., Harper, J.M. *et al.* (1974) Periurethral teflon injection for urinary incontinence. *Journal of Urology,* **111,** 180–3.
45. Caione, P., Lais, A., De Gennaro, M. *et al.* (1993) Glutaraldehyde cross-linked bovine collagen in exstrophy/epispadias complex. *Journal of Urology,* **150**, 631–3.
46. Scott, F.B., Bradley, W.E. and Timm, G.W. (1974) Treatment of urinary incontinence by an implantable prosthetic urinary sphincter. *Journal of Urology,* **112**, 75–80.
47. Light, J.K. (1985) The artificial urinary sphincter in children. *Urologic Clinics of North America,* **12**, 103–9.
48. Gonzalez, R., Nguyen, D.H., Koleilat, N. *et al.* (1989) Compatibility of enterocystoplasty and the artificial urinary sphincter. *Journal of Urology,* **142**, 502–4.
49. Montague, D.K. (1992) The artificial urinary sphincter (AS 800): experience in 166 consecutive patients. *Journal of Urology,* **147**, 380–2.
50. Hendren, W.H. (1973) Reconstruction of previously diverted urinary tracts in children. *Journal of Paediatric Surgery,* **8**, 135–50.
51. Ahmed, S. and Boucaut, H.A.P. (1987) Urinary undiversion in 35 patients with neurogenic bladder and an ileal conduit. *Australian and New Zealand Journal of Surgery,* **57**, 753–61.
52. Mitchell, M.E. (1986) Use of bowel in undiversion. *Urologic Clinics of North America,* **13**, 349–59.
53. Sheldon, C.A. (1996) Urinary reconstruction (rather than diversion) for continence in difficult pediatric urologic disorders. *Seminars in Pediatric Surgery,* **5**, 8–15.
54. Diamond, D.A., Blight, A., Samuell, C.T. *et al.* (1991) Ammonia levels in paediatric

ureterosigmoidostomy patients: a screen for hyperammonaemia. *British Journal of Urology,* **67**, 541–4.

55. Nurse, D.E. and Mundy, A.R. (1989) Metabolic complications of cystoplasty. *British Journal of Urology,* **63**, 165–70.
56. Sheiner, J.R. and Kaplan, G.W. (1988) Spontaneous bladder rupture following enterocystoplasty. *Journal of Urology,* **140**, 1157–8.
57. Beseghi, U., Guys, J.M., DiBenedetto, V. *et al.* (1996) Metabolic consequences of sigmoidocystoplasty in children. *Pediatric Surgery International*, **11**, 150–2.
58. Woodhouse, C.R.J., Wagstaff, K.E., Hotham, K. *et al.* (1991) Metabolic consequences of enterocystoplasty. *British Journal of Urology,* **68**, 644–5.
59. Kosko, J.W., Kursh, E.D. and Resnick, M.I. (1986) Metabolic complications of urologic intestinal substitutes. *Urologic Clinics of North America*, **13**, 193–200.
60. Koch, M.O. and McDougal, W.S. (1985) The pathophysiology of hyperchloremic metabolic acidosis after urinary diversion through intestinal segments. *Surgery,* **98**, 561–70.
61. Lockhart, J.L., Davies, R., Persky, L. *et al.* (1994) Acid–base changes following urinary tract reconstruction for continent diversion and orthotopic bladder replacement. *Journal of Urology,* **152,** 338–42.
62. Gleeson, M.J., Cunnane, G. and Graiger, R. (1991) Spontaneous perforation of an augmented bladder. *British Journal of Urology,* **68**, 655.
63. Crane, J.M., Scherz, H.S., Billman, G.F. *et al.* (1991) Ischemic necrosis: a hypothesis to explain the pathogenesis of spontaneously ruptured enterocystoplasty. *Journal of Urology,* **146**, 141–4.
64. Buson, H., Diaz, D.C., Manivel, J.C. *et al.* (1993) The development of tumors in experimental gastro-enterocystoplasty. *Journal of Urology,* **150**, 730–3.
65. Mundy, A.R. and Nurse, D.E. (1992) Calcium balance, growth and skeletal mineralisation in patients with cystoplasties. *British Journal of Urology,* **69**, 257–9.
66. Canning, D.A., Perman, J.A., Jeffs, R.D. *et al.* (1989) Nutritional consequences of bowel segments in the lower urinary tract. *Journal of Urology,* **142**, 509–11.
67. Filmer, R.B. and Spencer, J.R. (1990) Malignancies in bladder augmentations and intestinal conduits. *Journal of Urology,* **143**, 671–8.
68. Taskasaki, E., Murahashi, I., Toyoda, M. *et al.* (1983) Signet ring adenocarcinoma of ileal segment following ileocystoplasty. *Journal of Urology,* **130**, 562–3.
69. Golomb, J., Klutke, C.G., Lewin, K.J. *et al.* (1989) Bladder neoplasms associated with augmentation cystoplasty: report of two cases and literature review. *Journal of Urology,* **142**, 377–80.
70. Murray, K., Nurse, D.E. and Mundy, A.R. (1995) Malignant change in enterocystoplasty: a histochemical assessment. *Urology Research,* **23**, 21–5.
71. Palmer, L.S., Franco, I., Kogan, S.J. *et al.* (1993) Urolithiasis in children following augmentation cystoplasty. *Journal of Urology,* **150**, 726–9.
72. Nurse, D.E., McInerney, P.D., Thomas, P.J. *et al.* (1996) Stones in enterocystoplasties. *British Journal of Urology,* **77**, 684–7.
73. Moorcraft, J., DuBoulay, C.E.H., Isaacson, P. *et al.* (1983) Changes in the mucosa of colon conduits with particular reference to the risk of malignant change. *British Journal of Urology,* **55**, 185–8.
74. Davidsson, T., Carlen, B., Bak-Jensen, E. *et al.* (1996) Morphologic changes in intestinal mucosa with urinary contact – effects of urine or disuse? *Journal of Urology,* **156**, 226–32.
75. Sinaiko, E. (1956) Artificial bladder from segment of stomach and study of effect of urine on gastric secretion. *Surgery, Gynecology and Obstetrics*, **102**, 433–8.
76. Sinaiko, E.S. (1960) Artificial bladder from gastric pouch. *Surgery, Gynecology and Obstetrics,* **111**, 155–62.
77. Coffey, R.C. (1911) Physiologic implantation of the severed ureter or common bile duct into the intestine. *Journal of the American Medical Association,* **56**, 397–403.
78. Stamey, T.A. (1956) The pathogenesis and implications of the electrolyte imbalance in ureterosigmoidostomy. *Surgery, Gynecology and Obstetrics*, **103**, 736–41.
79. Ferris, D.O. and Odel, H.M. (1950) Electrolyte pattern of the blood after bilateral ureterosigmoidostomy. *Journal of the American Medical Association*, **142**, 634–9.

80. Bricker, E.M. (1952) Functional results of small intestinal segments on bladder substitute following pelvic evisceration. *Surgery,* **32**, 372–5.
81. Martin, D.C., Schultz, J.I. and Goodwin, W.E. (1962) Experimental autografting of gastric mucosa in the urinary tract to maintain persistent acid urine. *Journal of Urology,* **87**, 739–41.
82. Leong, C.H. and Ong, G.B. (1972) Gastrocystoplasty in dogs. *Australian and New Zealand Journal of Surgery*, **41**, 272–9.
83. Leong, C.H. (1978) Use of the stomach for bladder replacement and urinary diversion. *Annals of the Royal College of Surgeons,* **60**, 283–9.
84. Lim, S.T.K., Lam, S.K., Lee, N.W. *et al.* (1983) Effects of gastrocystoplasty and serum gastrin levels on gastric acid secretion. *British Journal of Surgery,* **70**, 275–7.
85. Tiffany, P., Vaughan, E.D. Jr, Marion, D. *et al.* (1986) Hypergastrinemia following antral gastrocystoplasty. *Journal of Urology,* **136**, 692–5.
86. Karow, W.F. and Thompson, I.M. (1969) Ureterogastrosigmoidostomy. *Surgery Forum*, **20**, 538–40.
87. Kennedy, H.A., Adams, M.C., Mitchell, M.E, *et al.* (1988) Chronic renal failure and bladder augmentation: stomach versus sigmoid colon in the canine model. *Journal of Urology,* **140**, 1138–40.
88. Adams, M.C., Mitchell, M.E. and Rink, R.C. (1988) Gastrocystoplasty: an alternative solution to the problem of urological reconstruction in the severely compromised patient. *Journal of Urology,* **140**, 1152–6.
89. Klee, L.W., Hoover, D.M., Mitchell, M.E. *et al.* (1990) Long term effects of gastrocystoplasty in rats. *Journal of Urology,* **144**, 1283–7.
90. Piser, J.A., Mitchell, M.E., Kulb, T.B. *et al.* (1987) Gastrocystoplasty and colocystoplasty in canines: the metabolic consequences of acute saline and acid loading. *Journal of Urology,* **138**, 1009–13.
91. Vaughan, E.D. and Tiffany, P. (1988) The use of gastrocystoplasty. *Dialogues in Pediatric Urology,* **11**, 6–9.
92. Ortiz, V. and Goldenberg, S. (1995) Hypergastrinemia following gastrocystoplasty in rats. *Urology Research*, **23**, 361–3.
93. Reinberg, Y., Manivel, J.C., Froemming, C. *et al.* (1992) Perforation of the gastric segment of an augmented bladder secondary to peptic ulcer disease. *Journal of Urology,* **148**, 369–71.
94. Nguyen, D.H., Bain, M.A., Salmonson, K.L. *et al.* (1993) The syndrome of dysuria and hematuria in pediatric urinary reconstruction with stomach. *Journal of Urology,* **150**, 707–9.
95. Gold, B.D., Bhoopalam, P.S., Reifen, R.M. *et al.* (1992) Gastrointestinal complications of gastrocystoplasty. *Archives of Diseases in Childhood,* **67**, 1272–6.
96. Gosalbez, R., Woodard, J.R., Broecker, B.H. *et al.* (1993) Metabolic complications of the use of stomach for urinary reconstruction. *Journal of Urology,* **150**, 710–12.
97. Sheldon, C.A., Gilbert, A., Wacksman, J. *et al.* (1995) Gastrocystoplasty: technical and metabolic characteristics of the most versatile childhood bladder augmentation modality. *Journal of Pediatric Surgery*, **30**, 283–8.
98. Dykes, E.H. and Ransley, P.G. (1992) Gastrocystoplasty in children. *British Journal of Urology,* **69**, 91–5.
99. Sanni-Bankole, R., Masson, J., Di Benedetto, V. *et al.* (1995) Gastrocystoplasty in the tretament of bladder exstrophy. *European Journal of Paediatric Surgery,* **5**, 342–7.
100. Sumfest, J.M. and Mitchell, M.E. (1994) Gastrocystoplasty in children. *European Urology,* **25,** 89–93.
101. Bogaert, G.A., Mevorach, R.A. and Kogan, B.A. (1994) Urodynamic and clinical follow-up of 28 children after gastrocystoplasty. *British Journal of Urology,* **74**, 469–75.
102. Di Benedetto, V., Beseghi, U., Bagnara, V. *et al.* (1996) The use of gastrocystoplasty in patients with bladder exstrophy. *Pediatric Surgery International,* **11**, 252–5.
103. Gosalbez, R., Woodard, J.R., Broecker, B.H. *et al.* (1993) The use of stomach in pediatric urinary reconstruction. *Journal of Urology,* **150**, 438–40.
104. Ngan, J.H.K., Lau, J.L.T., Lim, S.T.K. *et al.* (1993) Long-term results of antral gastrocystoplasty. *Journal of Urology,* **149**, 731–4.
105. Shoemaker, W.C. (1955) Reversed seromuscular grafts in urinary tract reconstruction. *Journal of Urology,* **74**, 453–75.
106. Shoemaker, W.C. and Marucci, H.D. (1955) The experimental use of seromuscular grafts in bladder reconstruction. *Journal of Urology*, **73**, 314–21.

107. Grotzinger, P., Shoemaker, W.C., Ulin, A.W. *et al.* (1954) The use of inverted seromuscular grafts from the ileum and colon for reconstruction of the urinary bladder. *Annals of Surgery*, **140**, 832–8.
108. Neuhof, H. (1917) Fascia transplantation into visceral defects. *Surgery, Gynecology and Obstetrics*, **24**, 383–7.
109. Campbell, E.W. (1957) Reconstruction of the bladder with a seromuscular graft. *Journal of Urology,* **78**, 236–41.
110. Martin, L.S.J. (1959) Uroepithelial lined ileal segment as a bladder replacement: experimental observations and brief review of literature. *Journal of Urology,* **82**, 633–49.
111. Blandy, J.P. (1964) The feasibility of preparing an ideal substitute for the urinary bladder. *Annals of the Royal College of Surgeons*, **35**, 287–311.
112. Blandy, J.P. (1961) Ileal pouch with transitional epithelium and anal sphincter as a continent urinary reservoir. *Journal of Urology,* **86**, 749–67.
113. Oesch, I. (1988) Neourothelium in bladder augmentation. *European Journal of Urology,* **14,** 328–9.
114. Motley, R.C., Montgomery, B.T., Zollman, P.E. *et al.* (1990) Augmentation cystoplasty utilizing de-epithelialized sigmoid colon: a preliminary study. *Journal of Urology,* **143**, 1257–60.
115. Salle, J.L., Fraga, J.C.S., Lucid, A. *et al.* (1990) Seromuscular enterocystoplasty in dogs. *Journal of Urology,* **144**, 454–6.
116. Badiola de, F., Manivel, J.C., and Gonzalez, R. (1991) Seromuscular enterocystoplasty in rats. *Journal of Urology,* **146**, 559–62.
117. Dewan, P.A., Lorenz, C., Stefanek, W. *et al.* (1994) Urothelial lined colocystoplasty in a sheep model. *European Journal of Urology*, **26**, 240–6.
118. Cheng, E., Rento, R., Grayhack, J.T. *et al.* (1994) Reversed seromuscular flaps in the urinary tract in dogs. *Journal of Urology,* **152,** 2252–7.
119. Haselhuhn, G.D., Kropp, K.A., Keck, R.W. *et al.* (1994) Photochemical ablation of intestinal mucosa for bladder augmentation. *Journal of Urology,* **152**, 2267–71.
120. Niku, S.D., Scherz, H.C., Stein, P.C. *et al.* (1995) Intestinal de-epithelialisation and augmentation cystoplasty: an animal model. *Urology,* **46**, 36–9.
121. Dewan, P.A., Stefanek, W. and Lorenz, C. (1995) Autoaugmentation gastrocystoplasty and demucosalised gastrocystoplasty in a sheep model. *Urology,* **45**, 291–5.
122. Frey, P., Lutz, N. and Leuba, A-L. (1996) Augmentation cystoplasty using pedicled and de-epithelialised gastric patches in the mini-pig model. *Journal of Urology,* **156**, 608–13.
123. Pompino, H-J., Loeffler, W. and Oerthel-Haid, D. (1973) The neurogenic bladder; an experimental study. *Progress in Pediatric Surgery,* **5**, 135–61.
124. Huggins, C.B. (1930) The formation of bone under the influence of epithelium of the urinary tract. *Archives of Surgery*, **22**, 377–408.
125. Mau, H. (1980) Die neurogene Blase – tierexperimentelle Untersuchungen zur Restauration der Blasenfunktion, Habilitationsschrift, Humboldt-Universität zu Berlin; 1.
126. Cartwright, P.C. and Snow, B.W. (1989) Bladder autoaugmentation: partial detrusor excision to augment the bladder without use of bowel. *Journal of Urology,* **142**, 1050–3.
127. Cartwright, P.C. and Snow, B.W. (1988) Partial detrusorectomy: augmenting the pediatric bladder without bowel. *Journal of Urology,* **139** Part 2, 234A, 287.
128. Moorhead, J.D. (1991) Detrusorectomy: autoaugmentation by a different name. *Dialogues in Pediatric Urology*, **14**, 4–5.
129. Gordon, E., Malone, P.R., Duffy, P.G. *et al.* (1991) The place of autocystoplasty in the management of the neuropathic bladder. *British Journal of Urology (Abstract),* **68**, 644–8.
130. Stothers, L., Johnson, H., Arnold, W. *et al.* (1994) Bladder autoaugmentation by vesicomyotomy in the pediatric neurogenic bladder. *Urology*, **44**, 110–13.
131. Ahmed, S. (1995) Bladder autoaugmentation (partial detrusor excision) for postoperative vesicoureteric reflux in a patient with posterior urethral valves. *Pediatric Surgery International*, **10**, 418–19.
132. Cartwright, P.C. and Snow, B.W. (1989) Bladder autoaugmentation: early clinical experience. *Journal of Urology,* **142**, 505–8.
133. Kennelly, M.J., Gormley, E.A. and McGuire, E.J. (1994) Early clinical experience with adult bladder auto-augmentation. *Journal of Urology,* **152**, 303–6.

134. Snow, B.W. and Cartwright, P.C. (1996) Bladder autoaugmentation. *Urologic Clinics of North America*, **23**, 323–31.
135. Morecroft, J.A., Searles, J. and MacKinnon, A.E. (1996) Detrusorectomy with Mitrofanoff stoma. *European Journal of Pediatric Surgery*, **6**(Suppl. I), 30–1.
136. Poppas, D.P., Uzzo, R.G., Britanisky, R.G. *et al.* (1996) Laparoscopic laser assisted auto-augmentation of the pediatric neurogenic bladder: early experience with urodynamic follow-up. *Journal of Urology*, **155**, 1057–60.
137. Dewan, P.A. and Byard, R.W. (1993) Autoaugmentation gastrocystoplasty in a sheep model. *British Journal of Urology,* **72**, 56–9.
138. Dewan, P.A., Lorenz, C. and Byard, R.W. (1993) Autoaugmentation gastrocystoplasty: the initial clinical experience. *British Journal of Urology* **74**, 460–4.
139. Dewan, P.A. and Stefanek, W. (1994) Autoaugmentation colocystoplasty. *Pediatric Surgery International*, **9**, 526–8.
140. Gonzalez, R., Buson, H., Reid, C. *et al.* (1995) Seromuscular colocystoplasty lined with urothelium: experience with 16 patients. *Urology*, **45**, 124–9.
141. Lima, S.V.C., Araujo, L.A.P., Vilar, F.O. *et al.* (1995) Nonsecretory sigmoid cystoplasty: experimental and clinical results. *Journal of Urology,* **153**, 1651–4.
142. Nguyen, D.H., Mitchell, M.E., Horowitz, M. *et al.* (1996) Demucosalised augmentation gastrocystoplasty with bladder autoaugmentation in pediatric patients. *Journal of Urology,* **156**, 206–9.
143. Garibay, J.T., Manivel, J.C. and Gonzalez, R. (1996) Effect of seromuscular colocystoplasty lined with urothelium and partial detrusorectomy on a new canine model of reduced bladder capacity. *Journal of Urology,* **154**, 903–6.
144. Dewan, P.A. and Lorenz, C. (1994) Bladder incorporation of large paraureteric diverticula: diverticulocystoplasty. *Australian and New Zealand Journal of Surgery,* **64**, 731–4.
145. Rittenberg, M.H., Hulbert, W.C., Snyder, H.M. and Duckett, J.W. (1900) Protective factors in posterior urethral valves. *Journal of Urology,* **140**, 993–6.
146. Churchill, B.M., Aliabadi, H., Landau, E.H. *et al.* (1992) Bladder reconstruction using ureteral augmentation constructed from megaureter. *Annual meeting of the Section of Urology,*American Academy of Peditrics, San Francisco No. 46 (abstract).
147. Dewan, P.A., Nicholls, E.A. and Goh, D.W. (1994) Ureterocystoplasty: an extraperitoneal, urothelial bladder augmentation technique. *European Urology,* **26**, 85–9.
148. Hitchcock, R.J.I., Duffy, P.G. and Malone, P.S. (1994) Ureterocystoplasty: the 'bladder' augmentation of choice. *British Journal of Urology,* **73**, 575–9.
149. Bellinger, M.F. (1993) Ureterocystoplasty: a unique method for vesical augmentation in children. *Journal of Urology,* **149**, 811–13.
150. Landau, E.H., Jayanthi, V.R., Khoury, A.E. *et al.* (1994) Bladder augmentation: ureterocystoplasty versus ileocystoplasty. *Journal of Urology,* **152**, 716–19.
151. Reinberg, Y., Allen, R.C., Vaughn, M. *et al.* (1995) Nephrectomy combined with lower abdominal extraperitoneal ureteral bladder augmentation in the treatment of children with the vesicoureteral reflux dysplasia syndrome. *Journal of Urology,* **153**, 177–9.
152. Churchill, B.M., Aliabadi, H., Landau, E.H. *et al.* (1993) Ureteral bladder augmentation. *Journal of Urology,* **150**, 716–20.
153. Schwarz, R. (1894) Della rigenerazione della vesica orinaria. *Rivista Veneta di Scienze Mediche* **20**, 484–92.
154. Perlmann, S. (1927) Demonstration zur Blasen-regeneration. *Zeitschrift für Urologie,* **21**, 621–3.
155. Tucci, P. and Haralambidis, G. (1963) Regeneration of the bladder: review of literature and case report. *Journal of Urology,* **90**, 193–8.
156. Neuhof, H. (1917) Fascia transplantation into visceral defects. *Surgery Gynecology and Obstetrics,* **24**, 383–427.
157. Kelami, A. (1975) Duraplasty of the urinary bladder – results after two to six years. *European Urology*, **1**, 178–81.
158. Jelly, O. (1970) Segmental cystectomy with peritoneoplasty. *Urology International*, **25**, 236–44.
159. Weingarten, J.L., Cromie, W.J. and Paty, R.J. (1990) Augmentation myoperitoneocystoplasty. *Journal of Urology,* **144**, 156–8.

160. Buyukunal, S.N.C., Kaner, G. and Celayir, S. (1989) An alternative treatment modality in closing bladder exstrophy: use of rectus abdominis flap – preliminary results in a rat model. *Journal of Pediatric Surgery,* **24**, 586–9.
161. Goldstein, M.B. and Dearden, L.C. (1966) Histology of omentoplasty of the urinary bladder in the rabbit. *Investigative Urology*, **3**, 460–9.
162. Novick, A.C., Straffon, R.A., Koshino, I. *et al.* (1978) Experimental bladder substitution using a biodegradable graft of natural tissue. *Journal of Biomedical Material Research*, **12**, 125–47.
163. Kambic, H., Kay, R., Chen, J-F. *et al.* (1992) Biodegradable pericardial implants for bladder augmentation: a 2.5 year study in dogs. *Journal of Urology,* **148**, 539–43.
164. Kelami, A., Dustmann, H.O., Luedtke-Handjery, A. *et al.* (1970) Experimental investigations of bladder regeneration using teflon-felt as a bladder wall substitute. *Journal of Urology,* **104**, 693–8.
165. Kaleli, A. and Ansell, J.S. (1984) The artificial bladder: a historical review. *Urology,* **24**, 423–8.
166. Stanley, T.H., Feminella, J.G., Priestley, J.B. *et al.* (1972) Subtotal cystectomy and prosthetic bladder replacement. *Journal of Urology,* **107**, 783–7.
167. Fishman, I.J., Flores, F.N., Scott, F.B. *et al.* (1987) Use of fresh placental membranes for bladder reconstruction. *Journal of Urology,* **138**, 1291–4.
168. Swinney, J. (1997) The use of prosthesis in the bladder. In Williams, D.I. and Chisholm, G.D. (eds.) *Scientific Foundations of Urology*. London, William Heinemann Medical Books Ltd: 353–5.
169. Sutherland, R.S., Baskin, L.S., Hayward, S.W. *et al.* (1996) Regeneration of bladder urothelium, smooth muscle, blood vessels and nerves into an acellular tissue matrix. *Journal of Urology,* **156**, 571–7.
170. Badylak, S.F., Lantz, G.C., Coffey, A. *et al.* (1989) Small intestinal submucosa as a large diameter vascular graft in the dog. *Journal of Surgical Research*, **47**, 74–7.
171. Kropp, B.P., Rippy, M., Badylak, S.F. *et al.* (1995) Small intestinal submucosa: urodynamic and histopathologic evaluation in long term canine bladder augmentation. *Journal of Urology,* **153**, 375A.
172. Kropp, B.P., Eppley, B.L., Prevel, C.D. *et al.* (1995) Experimental assessment of small intestinal submucosa as a bladder wall substitute. *Urology,* **46**, 396–400.
173. Kropp, B.P., Sawyer, B.D., Shannon, H.E. *et al.* (1996) Characterisation of small intestinal submucosa regenerated canine detrusor: assessment of reinnervation, in vitro compliance and contractility. *Journal of Urology,* **156,** 599–607.
174. Probst, E., Dahiya, R., Carrier, S. *et al.* (1997) Reproduction of functional smooth muscle tissue and partial bladder replacement. *British Journal of Urology,* **79**, 505–15.
175. Rheinwald, J.G. and Green, H. (1975) Serial cultivation of human epidermal keratocytes ; the formation of keratinizing colonies from single cells. *Cell*, **6**, 331–4.
176. Herz, F., Gazivoda, P., Papenhausen, P.R. *et al.* (1985) Normal human urothelial cells in culture. Subculture procedure, flow cytometric and chromosomal analyses. *Laboratory Investigations*, **53**, 571–4.
177. Johnson, M.D., Bryan, G.T. and Reznikoff, C.A. (1985) Serial cultivation of normal rat bladder epithelial cells in vitro. *Journal of Urology,* **133**, 1076–81.
178. Reznikoff, C.A., Loretz, L.J., Pesciotta, D.M. *et al.* (1987) Growth kinetics and differentiation in vitro of normal human uroepithelial cells on collagen gel substrates in defined medium. *Journal of Cell Physiology*, **131**, 285–301.
179. Hutton, K.A.R., Trejdosiewicz, L.K., Thomas, D.F.M. *et al.* (1993) Urothelial tissue culture for bladder reconstruction: an experimental study. *Journal of Urology,* **150**, 721–5.
180. Cilento, B.G., Freeman, M.R., Schneck, F.X. *et al.* (1994) Phenotypic and cytogenetic characterisation of human bladder urothelia expanded in vitro. *Journal of Urology*, 665–70.
181. Southgate, J., Hutton, K.A.R., Thomas, D.F.M. *et al.* (1994) Normal human urothelial cells in vitro: proliferation and induction of stratification. *Laboratory Investigations*, **71**, 583–94.
182. Petzoldt, J.L., Leigh, I.M., Duffy, P.G. *et al.* (1994) Culture and characterisation of human urothelium in vivo and in vitro. *Urology Research*, **22**, 67–74.
183. Smith, M.D., Shearer, M.G., Srivastava, S. *et al.* (1992) Quantitative evaluation of the growth of established cell lines on the surface of collagen, collagen composite and reconstituted basement membrane. *Urology Research*, **20**, 285–8.

184. Fujiyama, C., Masaki, Z. and Sugihara, H. (1995) Reconstruction of the urinary bladder mucosa in three-dimensional collagen gel culture: fibroblast–extracellular matrix interactions on the differentiation of transitional epithelial cells. *Journal of Urology,* **153**, 2060–7.
185. Atala, A., Freeman, M.R., Vacanti, J.P. *et al.* (1993) Implantation in vivo and retrieval of artificial structures consisting of rabbit and human urothelium and human bladder muscle. *Journal of Urology,* **150**, 608–12.
186. Lorenz, C., Maier-Reif, K., Back, W. *et al.* (1996) Cultured urothelium in sheep bladder augmentation. *Pediatric Surgery International,* **11**, 456–61.
187. Merguerian, P., Chavez, D.R. and Hakim, S. (1994) Grafting of cultured urothelium and bladder mucosa into de-epithelialised segments of colon in rabbits. *Journal of Urology,* **152**, 671–4.
188. Schaefer, B.M., Lorenz, C., Back, W. *et al.* (1998) Autologous transplantation of urothelium into demucosalised gastrointestinal segments: evidence for epithelialisation and differentiation of in vitro expanded and transplanted urothelial cells. *Journal of Urology,* **159,** 284–90.
189. Atala, A. (1995) Tissue engineering in the urinary tract. *Dialogues in Pediatric Urology*, **18**, 6–8.

2

Dilatation of the external urethral sphincter and its effect on the bladder

JOHN M PARK AND DAVID A BLOOM

INTRODUCTION

In English usage, the word dilatation preceded dilation and was first recorded in 1386 in Geoffrey Chaucer's *Man of Law's Tale*.[1] The term at the time referred to the practice of amplifying, enlarging or expanding on a topic. Dilatation, or dilation as it became known in shorter form, was well established in ancient medical practice, long before the Middle Ages. The *Sushruta Samhita*, for example, documented Indian healers around 1000 BC dilating urethral strictures.[2] Over the millennia that intervened, urethral dilation remained an enduring necessity in instances of stricture disease. Semantically, whether we use the term 'dilation' or 'dilatation' is inconsequential, although the shorter form may enjoy the wider usage.

Modern genitourinary surgery emerged at the start of the twentieth century as a distinct surgical specialty, when, with its new cystoscopic and radiological tools, urinary tract infection, vesicoureteral reflux, and enuresis became subjects of urological inquiry. Obstructive etiologies were postulated, and urethral dilation, performed expeditiously during the cystoscopic portion of investigation, was a natural consequence. Pediatric urology was firmly established as a subspecialty by 1960, and urodynamic investigations promptly ruled out an obstructive etiology in most of the common conditions. Furthermore, refined pediatric urologic algorithms for reflux, infection, and voiding dysfunction eliminated the routine use of cystoscopy and the convenient context for urethral dilation in these children. For pediatric genitourinary specialists, urethral dilation reverted to its original application of correction of urethral stricture.

One of the phenomenal accomplishments of twentieth-century medicine has been the salvage of infants with myelomeningocele, and their opportunity for functional lives with dignity and the preservation of renal function. In 1969, Perlmutter had commented in Matson's textbook of pediatric neurosurgery: 'It is widely recognised that the commonest causes of morbidity and mortality among children with spina bifida who survive beyond the first three years of life, are pyelonephritis and renal failure.'[3]

At one great center for pediatric urology, a clinician with an elegantly prepared mind made an important observation in his myelomeningocele population. Herbie Johnston in Liverpool, England, noted that a small percentage of myelomeningocele patients had urinary retention, upper-tract changes, and clinical problems early in infancy. Curiously, most of the children in this problematic subset were girls. Johnston empirically dilated the urethra 'to its limits of distention' and thereby resolved the clinical problems and stabilized or improved the upper tracts. His paper in 1971 received little attention.[4] The following year, Shochat and Perlmutter reported similar results in two girls with severe hydroureteronephrosis following closure of the open myelodysplastic defect.[5]

McGuire's concept of the leak-point pressure (LPP) revolutionized the management of myelomeningocele patients by providing a link between the lower urinary-tract storage parameters and upper tract safety.[6] At the University of Michigan in Ann Arbor, Johnston's technique of urethral dilation was utilized to lower the LPP in a select group of myelomeningocele patients with high LPPs.[7] Without question, urethral dilation reduced the LPP and provided a satisfactory alternative to vesicostomy.

Bladder compliance in myelodysplasia had been a topic of great interest in Ann Arbor.[8] Therefore, it seemed logical to look at compliance in bladders some years after urethral dilation. It was curious that the subgroup of children undergoing urethral dilation, who had been selected by virtue of their high LPPs, was similar to Johnston's patients in terms of female predominance and percentage of the entire myelomeningocele population (5%). Longitudinal measurements of bladder pressure–volume relationships revealed durable improvement in compliance in the initial report of 1–5-year outcome in 1990.[9] Those data suggested that noncompliant bladders are acquired because of high outlet resistance. Accordingly, we postulated that early intervention might improve long-term bladder storage characteristics. Analysis of these same patients, 10 years later, supports that hypothesis.

PHILOSOPHY OF MANAGEMENT

At the University of Michigan, patients with myelomeningocele, and with other neuropathic voiding dysfunctions such as traumatic spinal cord injury, are followed with a surveillance program that consists of periodic genitourinary imaging and urodynamic evaluations. Initial studies typically include renal ultrasonography, cystometrography (CMG), and voiding cystourethrography (VCUG). Ultrasonography provides the baseline for comparison to future studies that might show renal growth as well as morphologic stability or change. VCUG displays bladder shape, bladder neck patency, and vesicoureteral reflux. Trabeculation and diverticula formation of the bladder wall indicate previous response to obstruction and high outlet resistance. The configurations of bladder neck and proximal urethra are indicative of sphincteric competence. Surveillance cystometrics monitor the detrusor storage function in terms of capacity and compliance. The success of clean intermittent catheterization (CIC) programs, upon which many myelomeningocele patients rely to empty the bladder, depends largely upon the low-pressure, high-compliance storage reservoir. The LPP represents the worst-case scenario in terms of bladder storage pressure. In the management of myelomeningocele patients on CIC, it becomes obvious that the LPP is somewhat of a misnomer, particularly if no leakage occurs. The LPP concept remains operative and valid, but perhaps a better description of what we intend to measure in these instances is the maximum typical storage pressure. We may come to realize that a high pressure should be present for only a small fraction of a 24-hour time interval. In someone with a normal bladder, storage pressures should be less than 10 to 15 cmH_20 and are exceeded only perhaps six times a day for less than 1 minute at a time during micturition. If we double these physiologic parameters, to 30 cmH_20 for 12 minutes, then we might define a deleterious storage condition as one with a pressure of 30 cmH_20 for more than 0.8% of a 24–hour period. This is a far cry from our sense of a safe situation when chronic storage conditions are less than 40 cmH_20. The origin of the number '40' was simply McGuire's observation that clinical, morphological and functional deterioration of the urinary tract was a readily observed consequence of chronic bladder pressures at or above 40 cmH_20. That observation hardly implies that a pressure maintained at 30 cmH_20 is good.

When LPPs or, more specifically the typical ambient bladder storage pressures are deemed unsafe, anticholinergic agents are utilized initially, along with adjustment of catheterization intervals. Urethral dilation is introduced when elevated LPP (storage pressure) and compliance do not improve. Thus, urethral dilation is an alternative to vesicostomy and an intermediate measure of intervention between pharmacological therapy and augmentation cystoplasty. As will be shown, urethral dilation alone has been adequate in improving the overall storage function in a small subset of patients, protecting upper-tract integrity and improving continence.

OPERATIVE TECHNIQUE

We currently perform urethral dilation under anesthesia. Other procedures are typically performed at the same time, such as cystoscopy, bladder irrigation, and disimpaction of hard stools. In female patients under 6–8 years of age, urethral sounds of up to 38 FG are adequate. Older patients may require Hegar dilators (up to No. 18). In male patients, dilation is more difficult because it must be performed through a perineal urethrostomy or with balloon distention under fluoroscopic control. Like Johnston and Kathel, we found a female predominance (almost 90%) among myelomeningocele patients requiring urethral dilation. The region of dilation is at the external urethral sphincter, which spans the membranous urethra on urethrogram and the zone of maximal urethral closure pressure on urethral pressure profilometry. Our goal is to dilate and stretch that area of striated muscle to its limits of distension. In females, modest resistance is felt at around 28 FG to 30 FG. Once past this point, however, the urethra can be smoothly dilated up to 36–38 FG with minimal resistance. It is easy imme-

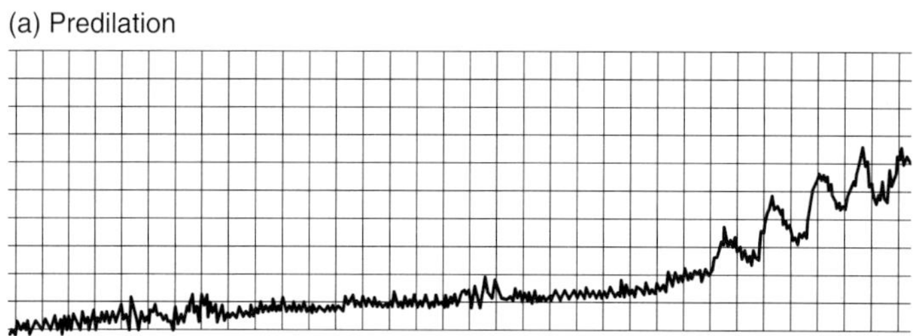

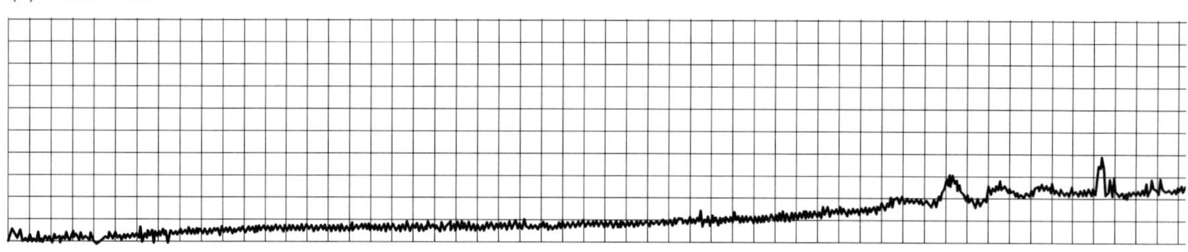

Figure 2.1 *An example of dramatic improvement in leak-point pressure (LPP) and overall storage characteristics after urethral dilation. This 4-year-old female patient with lumbar myelomeningocele had a LPP exceeding 60 cmH_2O and bladder capacity less than 100 ml. The external urethral sphincter was dilated to 34F. Urodynamic tracing 6 months after dilation shows a reduction of LPP to 22 cmH_2O, as well as improved capacity and compliance.*

diately to check the LPP with a water manometer in the operating room, to be certain that the goal of lowering the LPP has been met. Urethroscopy immediately after dilation is surprisingly unremarkable, and the membranous urethra typically has a mild degree of erythema and edema. A small epithelial tear at the urethral meatus is common after dilation, but excessive bleeding is unusual. We do not routinely leave an indwelling catheter, and patients are restarted on CIC immediately.

Even though lowered LPP is evident in cystometrograms (CMGs) performed immediately after urethral dilation, improved storage characteristics in terms of capacity and compliance are not usually seen for several weeks (Fig. 2.1). This suggests that improvement in bladder storage function after urethral dilation is a gradual, adaptive response to the lowered outlet resistance, rather than an immediate effect of urethral dilation. Patients are therefore brought back approximately 4 to 6 weeks after dilation for a follow-up CMG. If adequate improvements in LPP and compliance are achieved, patients are re-evaluated 6–12 months later. If the improvement in urodynamic parameters is inadequate and storage pressures are still deemed unsafe, urethral dilation is repeated. Failure to improve after a trial of urethral dilation generally indicates the need for conventional surgical alternatives, such as vesicostomy or augmentation cystoplasty.

OUTCOME

Among more than 350 myelomeningocele patients managed at the University of Michigan Pediatric Urology Clinic over 15 years, 18 patients (16 female, two male) with elevated bladder storage pressures have undergone urethral dilation and been followed for at least 6 years (mean follow-up 9.1 year). The average age at first dilation was 2.9 years (range 1 week to 9 years). Eight have been followed since the neonatal period. A total of 38 dilations were performed in these patients, with an average of 2.1 dilations per patient. Seven required only one dilation. Predilation LPP averaged 55.7 cmH_2O, while at the most recent follow-up, the average LPP was 30.0 cmH_2O ($p<0.01$, paired t-test). In terms of capacity (defined as the bladder volume at which passive leakage occurs during filling), predilation capacity averaged 106.6 ml, and at the most recent follow-up it was 242.8 ml ($p<0.01$). The interval increase in bladder capacity may reflect the patients' overall somatic growth, as well as the effect of urethral dilation. Nevertheless, these high-risk patients may have lost their ability to appropriately increase bladder capacity with growth, had they not been treated with urethral dilation. Compliance, which is the inverse of bladder stiffness during filling and storage, describes a bladder's pressure–volume relationship. While one may subjectively interpret a given filling curve as having 'good-or-bad' compliance, there is currently no consensus in terms of further description. The bladder is an organ of great adaptive response to a wide range of volumes, maintaining a constant, low pressure. Compliance is an instantaneous phenomenon that may vary from the initial through to the terminal phases of filling.[8] The initial compliance varies significantly among patients and appears to predict the bladder's overall storage function for patients on CIC, whereas the terminal compliance may be more important in patients relying on passive leakage. When the response to urethral dilation was analyzed in terms of initial and terminal compliance calculations (Fig. 2.2) a significant and durable improvement was noted for both. At predilation, initial and terminal compliance values were 13.5 ml/cmH_2O and 0.6 ml/cmH_2O respectively, while at the most recent follow-up, they were 20.8 ml/cmH_2O and 1.6 ml/cmH_2O ($p<0.01$ for both). With respect to LPP, capacity, and compliance, the improvements after urethral dilation appeared to be durable over a long-term follow-up.

Upper-tract status remained stable in all patients. This is in contrast to McGuire's original report describing the prognostic relevance of elevated LPP, wherein greater than 80% of patients with LPP exceeding 40 cmH_2O developed upper-tract deterioration. Thus, it appears that the duration of the high-storage pressures has greater prognostic significance than the pressures alone.

In terms of continence, seven patients (39%) reported wetness between catheterizations (although they were not bothered by it, and were not interested in further intervention), whereas the rest were either dry or minimally damp (requiring less than one pad

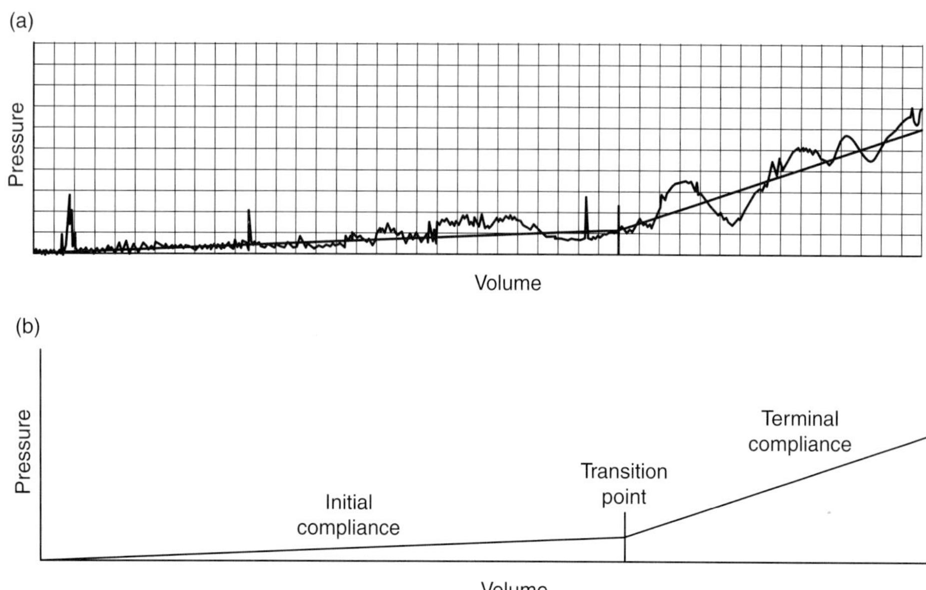

Figure 2.2 *Calculation of initial and terminal compliance. The point of transition is arbitrarily chosen in the cystometric tracing where a flatter, initial portion of the curve changes to a steeper, terminal portion. Slopes are then calculated in these regions as change in volume (ml) per change in pressure (cmH_2O). In our study of myelomeningocele patients who were managed with urethral dilation, one investigator chose the transition points in all tracings to minimize any interobserver variability.*

per day) between catheterizations. It has been suggested that lowering of outlet resistance by urethral dilation might jeopardize the continence mechanism. Our contention is that the high outlet resistance offered by the neurologically denervated external urethral sphincter provides no meaningful sphincteric function, and that it only stands to further compromise the eventual continence by worsening capacity and compliance over time. In analyzing these patients, it became apparent that lowering the LPP by urethral dilation did not adversely affect continence outcome. The average LPP for wet patients was 30.1 cmH_2O, while that for dry/damp patients was 30.8 cmH_2O (the difference was not statistically significant). In fact, the parameters that best correlated with the continence outcome were the response to urethral dilation in terms of capacity (146 ml vs. 322 ml, $p<0.01$) and compliance (7.7 ml/cmH_2O vs. 22.8 ml/cmH_2O, $p<0.01$, for initial compliance; 0.6 ml/cmH_2O vs. 2.2 ml/cmH_2O, $p<0.01$, for terminal compliance). The lowering of outlet resistance by urethral dilation probably facilitated continence by improving bladder storage function.

All but one patient, so far, have been managed without augmentation cystoplasty or diversion. This particular patient underwent ileal enterocystoplasty 8 years after the initial urethral dilation. She was first seen in our clinic as a 6 year old, and the baseline CMG revealed a LPP of 45 cmH_2O at 120 ml of hypertonic filling. At that time, she already had a bilateral vesicoureteral reflux (grade V on the left and grade I on the right). Renal ultrasonography revealed mild pelvicaliectasis on the left, with normal parenchymal thickness on both. With the first urethral dilation, LPP was lowered from 45 cmH_2O to 23 cmH_2O. This patient required three more dilations for recurrent elevation of her LPP at the ages of 9, 10, and 13 years. Her upper tract remained stable, and subsequent ultrasonography revealed an appropriate growth in both kidneys with a stable, mild pelvicaliectasis on the left. In terms of continence, she reported only dampness, requiring only one pad a day. Recurrent urinary-tract infections, in spite of antibiotic prophylaxis, a good catheterization routine and bowel control, became troublesome during the latter years of follow-up (two to three febrile infections a year). Her LPPs ranged consistently between 25 and 30 cmH_2O, with the capacity exceeding 300 ml. Despite the above urodynamic findings, we felt that the overall hypertonicity of the initial phase of the filling curve was contributing to the persistent reflux and recurrent urinary-tract infections. After ileocystoplasty, the baseline storage pressures fell to 15 cmH_2O with a capacity well exceeding 400 ml. Without ureteral reimplantation, postoperative cystogram revealed a resolution of reflux. She still requires antibiotic prophylaxis; however, she has not experienced any further episodes of febrile infections.

HOW BLADDER COMPLIANCE IS MAINTAINED: LESSONS LEARNED

It is well documented that elevated bladder pressures resulting from high outlet resistance during storage and elimination of urine lead to upper-tract deterioration. Furthermore, other lower urinary-tract complications, such as infection and incontinence, have also been linked to elevated bladder pressures. Although CIC usually achieves the goal of low-pressure urine emptying in most patients with neuropathic voiding dysfunctions, its ultimate success is largely dependent upon the bladder's ability to store urine under low, safe pressures.

Our experience of using urethral dilation in a subset of high-pressure, poor-compliance myelomeningocele patients has provided important clues regarding the role of the external urethral sphincter in determining the bladder's overall ability to store urine. One such observation was that bladder compliance is the critical link between upper urinary-tract status and outlet resistance. When the bladder is forced to empty itself against a high outlet resistance, it will gradually lose its storage capability, manifested by a worsening compliance; and when the compliance becomes bad enough, the upper tracts will eventually suffer. Our original intent with external urethral sphincter dilation was simply to lower the bladder's 'pop-off' storage pressures, so that the upper tracts would be protected. External sphincter dilation has certainly achieved this goal in all our patients, but it also provided the additional benefit of improved compliance and overall storage function, which may have resulted in better continence and fewer urinary-tract infections. Continence is an end-result of complex interactions between detrusor (reservoir) and bladder-neck/rhabdosphincter (outlet resistance). Most patients with myelomeningocele have a variable degree of denervation to the bladder neck and external urethral sphincter, and the degree of continence is a direct reflection of detrusor function in terms of storage capability. Despite a significant lowering of outlet resistance (measured by a fall in LPPs), continence was excellent in the majority of our patients, and the key determining factor was response to external sphincter dilation in terms of improved capacity and compliance.

What then regulates the bladder's compliance? Both mechanical distensibility of the bladder wall – determined by smooth muscle and extracellular matrix content – and neural modulation of bladder tone play important roles. The bladder responds to an increased workload by an adaptive response of cellular proliferation and hypertrophy. Increased stromal cells (smooth muscle cells and fibroblasts) and deposition of extracellular matrix (collagen, fibronectin) probably contribute to the increased wall thickness and loss of distensibility.[10] This paradigm of proliferative response to increased workload is common to other organs. The heart, for example, seemed to undergo proliferative changes, similar to those of the bladder, when subjected to high outlet resistance.[11] Various genes are activated to synthesize cytokines and growth factors that direct these proliferative responses. When outlet resistance is lowered or eliminated, many of these changes will revert back toward the baseline. The bladder probably undergoes a similar cascade of molecular events and biochemical alterations when it too is subjected to high outlet resistance. By lowering the resistance with urethral dilation, we may be decreasing the workload for the bladder, restoring the proper homeostatic balance of bladder-wall components for optimal compliance.

Neurally mediated regulation of bladder contractility and tone also plays an important role in the maintenance of bladder compliance. When the nervous system input to the lower urinary tract is eliminated, both experimentally[12] and clinically,[13] the external urethral sphincter activity becomes fixed relative to bladder filling, and the filling curve becomes significantly hypertonic. The concept of the *guarding reflex*, proposed by R.C. Garry in 1959, describes a reciprocal relationship between the external urethral sphincter and bladder.[14] Filling is associated with a progressive increase in external urethral sphincter activity. Just prior to the onset of voiding contraction, the external sphincter becomes electrically silent and remains so throughout the duration of voiding contraction. When one attempts to halt the ongoing bladder contraction, the external sphincter forcefully contracts first, which is then followed by the disappearance of bladder activity. It is as if the bladder takes its cue for contraction or relaxation from the external urethral sphincter. Similarly, aberrant bladder contractions may be silenced by activation of the external urethral sphincter. In patients with traumatic spinal cord injury, for example, uninhibited bladder contractions can be suppressed by external sphincter dilation, as well as by activation of the bulbocavernosus reflex.[15] The external urethral sphincter's role in lower urinary-tract function may well be the bladder's 'on–off' switch for contraction and relaxation.[16] The degree of denervation contributing to the loss of neurally mediated compliance in myelodysplastic patients, is probably quite variable and difficult to estimate. It is possible, however, that part of the compliance deficiency in myelomeningocele patients may stem from inadequate neurally mediated bladder inhibition (guarding reflex). The external urethral sphincter dilation may alter the local neuromuscular environment near the external sphincter, 'augmenting' its guarding reflex.

CONCLUSIONS

The critical functions of the lower urinary tract are storage, continence, and effective emptying, all accomplished at safe intravesical pressures. The common denominator in the three critical functions and their dysfunction is the detrusor. A miracle of genetic engineering throughout the animal kingdom has achieved these goals, and yet allowed each species to express its own peculiarities of micturition. When the system goes awry, either through congenital anomaly, physical trauma or behavioral dysfunction, social and renal well-being are jeopardized.

REFERENCES

1. Bloom, D.A., Mory, R.N. and Hinman, F. Jr (1992) Dilation vs. dilatation: a brief history. *Journal of Urology*, **147**, 1682.
2. Das, S. (1983) Sushruta of India, the pioneer in the treatment of urethral stricture. *Surgery, Gynecology and Obstetrics*, **157**, 581.
3. Matson, D.D. (1969) *Neurosurgery of Infancy and Childhood*, 2nd edn. Springfield, IL, Charles C. Thomas.
4. Johnston, J.H. and Kathel, B.L. (1971) The obstructed neurogenic bladder in the newborn. *British Journal of Urology*, **43**, 206–10.
5. Shochat, S.J. and Perlmutter, A.D. (1972) Myelodysplasia with severe neonatal hydronephrosis; the value of urethral dilation. *Journal of Urology*, **107**, 146–8.
6. Wang, S.C., McGuire, E.J. and Bloom, D.A. (1988) A bladder pressure management system for myelodysplasia – clinical outcome. *Journal of Urology*, **140**, 1499–502.
7. Wang, S.C., McGuire, E.J. and Bloom, D.A. (1989) Urethral dilation in the management of urological complications of myelodysplasia. *Journal of Urology*, **142**, 1054–5.
8. Ghoneim, G.M., Bloom, D.A., McGuire, E.J. and Stewart, K.L. (1989) Bladder compliance in myelomeningocele children. *Journal of Urology*, **141**, 1404–6.
9. Bloom, D.A., Knechtel, J.M. and McGuire, E.J. (1990) Urethral dilation improves bladder compliance in children with myelomeningocele and high leak point pressures. *Journal of Urology*, **144**, 430–3.
10. Levin, R.M. Wein, A.J., Buttyan, R. *et al.* (1994) Update on bladder smooth muscle physiology. *World Journal of Urology*, **12**, 226–32.
11. Yamazaki, T., Komuro, I. and Yazaki, Y. (1995) Molecular mechanism of cardiac cellular

hypertrophy by mechanical stress (review). *Journal of Molecular Cell Cardiology,* **27,** 133–40.

12. McGuire, E.J. and Morrissey, S.G. (1982) The development of neurogenic vesicula dysfunction after experimental spinal cord injury or sacral rhizotomy in non-human primates. *Journal of Urology,* **128,** 1390–3.
13. Woodside, J.R. and McGuire, E.J. (1982) Detrusor hypertonicity as a late complication of a Wertheim hysterectomy. *Journal of Urology,* **127,** 1143–5.
14. Garry, R.C., Roberts, T.D.M. and Todd, J.K. (1959) Reflexes involving the external urethral sphincter in the cat. *Journal of Physiology,* **149,** 653–63.
15. Park, J.M., Wedemeyer, G. and Bloom, D.A. (1995) Suppression of uninhibited bladder contractions by stimulation of external urethral sphincter. Abstract. Presented at the American Academy of Pediatrics Meeting, San Francisco, CA.

3

Bladder stimulation and sacral rhizotomy

EARL Y CHENG AND WILLIAM E KAPLAN

INTRODUCTION

In light of many of the problems and complications associated with bladder reconstructive procedures, alternative methods of managing the neurogenic bladder which are less invasive than bladder augmentation are desirable. Two of these methods, intravesical transurethral bladder stimulation therapy and selective posterior rhizotomy, have been investigated. Preliminary results suggest that both of these therapies can be extremely successful in selected patients, and may serve as an alternative to augmentation cystoplasty. In this chapter, both of these treatment modalities are described in detail. Also, the advantages and disadvantages of their use in the treatment of the patient with a neurogenic bladder are discussed.

BLADDER STIMULATION

The use of intravesical transurethral bladder stimulation therapy in children with myelomeningocele and a neurogenic bladder was first described by Katona and Berenyi in Hungary in 1975.[1] Preliminary results from their first 100 patients demonstrated that spontaneous voiding along with acceptable continence could be achieved in over 70% of patients treated. Successful utilization of this therapy has also been demonstrated in adult patients with incomplete spinal cord injuries by Madersbacher *et al.*[2] Encouraged by these results, utilization of bladder stimulation therapy was first begun in the USA in 1984 at Children's Memorial Hospital (CMH) in Chicago. Since then, over 500 children with myelomeningocele and a neurogenic bladder have been treated with this novel therapy at CMH and at other centers across the USA. Despite extensive clinical experience, the physiological effects of bladder stimulation on bladder wall dynamics are just now beginning to be understood. Prognostic indicators for a successful result are also being identified. It is hoped that further experience with bladder stimulation will provide greater insight into the mechanism of action of this therapy, and enable better selection of patients who will benefit most from this treatment modality.

Bladder stimulation technique

The technique which is currently used at CMH is essentially the same as that described by Katona and Berenyi[1] with minor modifications. Initially, the patient is thoroughly evaluated and the goals, advantages, disadvantages, and potential complications of the therapy are discussed in detail with the patient and family. This discussion is important, because the therapy is labor intensive for all involved, and a clear understanding of the program is necessary if patient compliance and success are to occur. Once therapy is agreed upon, the patient has an initial urodynamic study, in which the bladder is catheterized and a slow-fill water cystometrogram (CMG) is performed. The bladder is filled at a rate of approximately 5% of estimated bladder capacity/minute. A leak-point pressure is determined at the first sign of leakage from the urethral meatus. At the end of the CMG, the bladder is emptied. This emptied volume is defined as the bladder capacity. The measured intravesical pressure at this volume is defined as the bladder capacity pressure. Following this initial CMG, the bladder is filled to half-capacity with normal saline via an electrocatheter. An initial 15–minute bladder observation period then follows, during which time no therapy is administered. This in turn is followed by a 90–minute therapy session. Observations made during this first evaluation are used in setting the parameters for future stimulation. Parameters which can be varied include intensity (current), frequency, pulse width (impulse duration), package, interval, and rise-time (Fig. 3.1). In general, a hypotonic bladder will receive an electrical package that is stronger and repeated more often than a hypertonic bladder. Children are initially treated with 20 separate 90–minute outpatient sessions (a series), during which time periodic adjustments will be made depending on the response of the bladder to stimulation. These periodic adjustments are crucial in achieving maximum benefit from this therapy. Following this first series, a CMG is performed and the bladder is allowed to rest for approximately 3 to 6 months. Upon returning, a repeat CMG is performed and a subsequent course of stimulation sessions (five to 15) is administered over 1 to 2 weeks. Further therapy is individualized to the patient's needs and responses.

Medications which may affect bladder dynamics (e.g., anticholinergics) are routinely discontinued a few days prior to urodynamic studies and during the course of bladder stimulation therapy. These medications are sometimes re-instituted between sessions, depending on the condition of the bladder of the individual patient. Nevertheless, all urodynamic studies are routinely performed off medications. In a few selected patients with very high storage pressures, medications are not discontinued during therapy for fear of upper-tract deterioration. In these patients, urodynamic studies are performed with the patients on the same doses of medications so that fair comparisons of studies and appropriate evaluation of progress can be made.

Results (Fig. 3.1)

When bladder stimulation therapy was first initiated at CMH, the primary goal was to create total

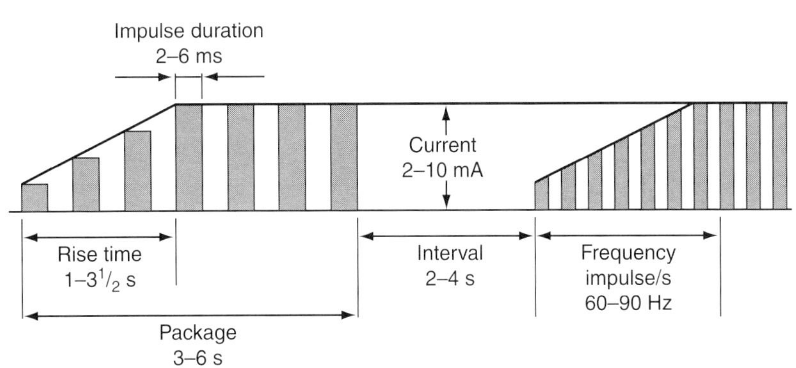

Figure 3.1 *Bladder stimulation parameters which can be varied include intensity (current), frequency, pulse width (impulse duration), package, interval, and rise time.*

conscious micturition control in the previously incontinent child who had little or no sensation of bladder filling. Early experience was positive, suggesting that success may be achieved in a fair number of patients. Evaluation of the first 62 patients treated with bladder stimulation at CMH revealed that 38% of patients (who underwent at least three series of treatments) were able to achieve satisfactory urinary continence and void with low pressure.[3,4] Patients who could respond to sensory signals of detrusor contraction during therapy, and could cooperate with biofeedback techniques, were most likely to establish improved urinary control. In the infant population, where participation in biofeedback techniques is not possible, goals of therapy are simply to decrease residual urine and improve functional bladder capacity. Further experience has shown that early improvement in bladder sensation, following the initiation of therapy, is a critical factor in determining if bladder stimulation will be successful. Nearly two-thirds of patients treated with bladder stimulation will achieve some sensation with either bladder filling or bladder contractions. The patients who develop improvement in bladder sensation early are also those who benefit most from the development of urinary control, volitional voiding, and/or improvement in bladder compliance. Although complete voluntary control of voiding is possible following therapy, review of long-term results from multiple institutions suggest that this is successfully achieved in only 15–20% of all children treated.

There are many theories as to how bladder stimulation works. The mechanism of action is not clear and has yet to be elucidated. However, as with neurologically intact individuals, the sensory limb of the detrusor response is a critical component in achieving normal bladder compliance and contractility. Recent data from experimental animals have further demonstrated the importance of afferent signals from the bladder, and parallels clinical observations that development of bladder sensation is a critical component in the response to therapy. In 1992, Ebner *et al.*[5] demonstrated in cats and rats that intravesical electrical stimulation directly activates bladder afferent mechanoreceptors, which leads to a reflexive activation of the detrusor muscle. These mechanoreceptors are in part responsible for the increase in sensation during bladder filling, and also provide the eventual drive for a bladder contraction. Repeated stimulation of this pathway, as is done in bladder stimulation, may therefore upgrade and 'awaken' dormant receptors present in the bladder of myelomeningocele patients. These experimental data provide preliminary evidence that bladder stimulation therapy physiologically alters bladder dynamics, and is not just a 'sham' treatment.

One of the most important beneficial effects of bladder stimulation, other than enhanced urinary control, is improved bladder compliance via an increase in bladder capacity and/or decrease in bladder storage pressures. With respect to bladder capacity and growth, it has been shown that the neurogenic bladder attains a growth pattern similar to that of a normal bladder following bladder stimulation therapy. In a comparative study of over 220 patients, it was found that the untreated myelomeningocele bladder had an average increase in bladder capacity of 15–20 cm^3/year, and that the capacity could be estimated from the equation:[6,7]

$$\text{bladder capacity} = 17\ cm^3 \times \text{age (years)} + 122\ cm^3$$

In contrast, the bladder treated with bladder stimulation had a yearly increase in capacity of 25–30 cm^3, and the bladder capacity could be estimated from the equation:

$$\text{bladder capacity} = 29\ cm^3 \times \text{age (years)} + 51\ cm^3$$

Interestingly, this estimation of bladder capacity is almost identical to the equation utilized to estimate capacity in the child with a normal bladder, as reported by Berger *et al.*:[8]

$$\text{bladder capacity} = 32\ cm^3 \times \text{age (years)} + 73\ cm^3$$

This illustrates that bladder stimulation functionally increases bladder capacity in the child with a neurogenic bladder, and initiates further bladder growth, which is nearly identical to the neurologically normal bladder (Fig. 3.2). This normalization of bladder growth translates clinically into improved bladder dynamics and compliance.

Intravesical bladder stimulation programs have now been developed at several institutions across the USA. Published individual results of some of the other centers' preliminary experience have not been entirely consistent with the encouraging findings

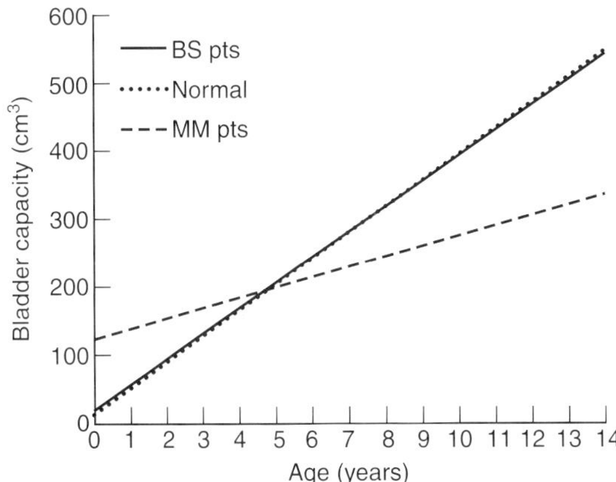

Figure 3.2 *Bladder growth in normal children (Normal), untreated myelomeningocele patients (MM Patients), and myelomeningocele patients treated with bladder stimulation (BS Patients). Note that the bladder growth in bladder stimulation patients is nearly identical to that of normal patients.*

observed at CMH with regard to success rates and patient satisfaction. Boone *et al.*[9] in 1992 reported on their experience with 36 children who were randomized prospectively to treatment and sham groups. They found no significant differences in bladder capacity between the two groups, and postulated that this may be due to irreversible histologic changes in the detrusor wall. The following year, Lyne and Bellinger[10] reported that five of 12 patients had sustained increases in bladder capacity following therapy. In 1994, Decter *et al.*[11] also reported an increase in age-adjusted bladder capacity in a similar percentage of patients, but also commented that they were not accepting new patients into their program because of a lack of significant alteration in patients' 'daily voiding routine' following therapy.

The reasons for the variability in success at different centers may be multifactorial. First, it must be emphasized that the administration of bladder stimulation therapy is operator dependent, and not just a 'set of directions.' Adjustments must be made during the course of therapy, which may substantially affect the overall result and clinical outcome. Given these reasons, there is a definite learning curve associated with this treatment modality. Aside from the method of administration, variability in success may also be related to the timing and number of urodynamic studies performed. One poor urodynamic study does not necessarily indicate a treatment failure. As Kaplan has previously noted,[7] improvement often occurs in a 'staircase'-like fashion: significant improvement, followed by some diminution, and then further improvement. In other words, if one observes diminution in bladder capacity but still continues therapy, this decrease will usually be transient, and further increase and improvement will eventually be seen. Therefore, it is the trend of improvement that is most important, not any single measurement of bladder dynamics. Persistence in therapy, when appropriate, is extremely important to achieve long-term success.

Although many variables exist which can influence the interpretation of results from this controversial treatment modality, the apparent incongruety of results observed at individual centers is a cause for concern. Recently, a large, multi-institutional trial was conducted, both to address this concern and to evaluate the efficacy of bladder stimulation to improve bladder compliance.[12] Institutions included in this study were chosen on the basis of the following criteria: (a) they had an active bladder stimulation program; and (b) the program was started in consultation with Children's Memorial Hospital in Chicago, following training at this institution. Centers were not excluded on the basis of results, patient population, experience, or number of patients treated. Institutions in this retrospective review included: Children's Memorial Hospital, Chicago, IL; St Michael's Hospital, Milwaukee, WI; Cardinal Glennon Children's Hospital, St Louis, MO; Children's Specialized Hospital, Mountainside, NJ; Arnold Palmer Hospital for Children and Women, Orlando, FL; Children's Developmental Center, Omaha, NE; Children's Hospital and Medical Center, Seattle, WA; University of Minnesota, Minneapolis, MN; Baylor Medical Center, Dallas, Texas; North Shore University Hospital, Manhasset, NY; and the Children's Hospital, Boston, MA.

All the charts from 568 patients undergoing bladder stimulation were evaluated. There were no preselection patient criteria utilized in this study. Three hundred and thirty-five of the 568 patients had adequate and accurate pre-treatment and post-treatment urodynamic studies, which included changes

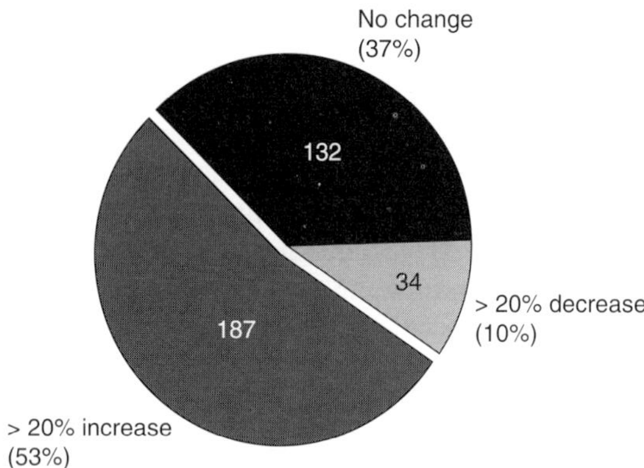

Figure 3.3 *Change in bladder capacity following bladder stimulation therapy in 353 patients from 11 separate institutions.*

in bladder capacity (BC) following treatment. Following bladder stimulation therapy, 53% of patients had an increased bladder capacity of more than 20%; 37% had no significant increase or decrease; and 10% had a decrease in bladder capacity of more than 20% (Fig. 3.3). In the 53% of patients who had a >20% increase in bladder capacity, the average volume increase following therapy was 102 cm^3 ($p<0.01$). This increase occurred over an average of 1.9 years. Since the average growth of the untreated myelomeningocele bladder is approximately 15–20 cm^3/year,[6] the observed 102 cm^3 increase over 1.9 years is far greater than the 30–40 cm^3 one would expect in untreated patients. This increase is also in excess of the 60–70 cm^3 expected in a normal child with a healthy bladder. Additionally, if the expected bladder capacity (EBC) is calculated using the formula EBC (cm^3) = (32 × age) + 73 15, this group of patients' percent EBC (actual BC/EBC) increased from a pretherapy value of 65% to 86% post-therapy ($p<0.01$) (Fig. 3.4). In other words, bladder stimulation therapy increased bladder capacity from 66% to 90% of normal capacity in this subset of patients.

To evaluate whether the increase in bladder capacity observed in these patients occurred at the expense of an increase in intravesical storage pressures, bladder capacity pressures (BCPs) were evaluated in this same subset of patients. Following therapy, 16% of patients lowered their BCP by >25%, while 74% had no significant change (Fig. 3.5). When these two groups are combined, one finds that 90% of patients either lowered or maintained their BCP in a safe range, while significantly increasing their bladder capacity. The average BCP in this combined group of patients was 28 cmH_2O, which is well below the 40 cmH_2O standard associated with upper-tract deterioration.[13] Unfortunately, 10% of patients with a significant increase in bladder capacity were also noted to have a >25% increase in their BCP. On further evaluation of these 17 patients, six were subsequently found to have a tethered cord, four eventually had a return of their BCP

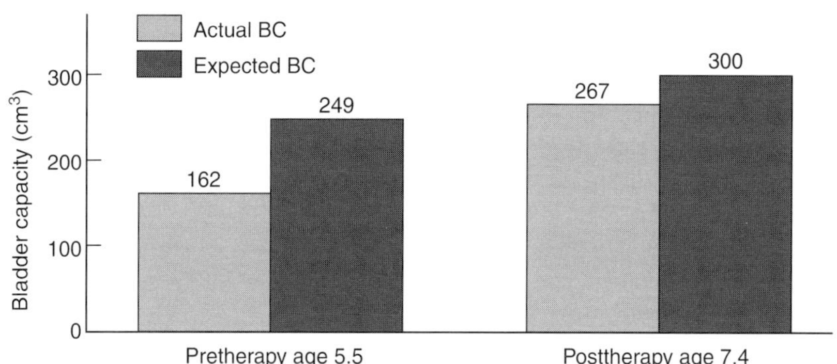

Figure 3.4 *Actual and expected bladder capacity in patients who responded to bladder stimulation with a >20% increase in BC. Actual BC increased from a pretherapy value of 162 cm^3 to 267 cm^3 post-therapy ($p<0.01$) over 1.9 years. When the actual BC is compared to the expected BC (EBC), the percent EBC (actual BC/EBC) increased from 65% (162/249) pretherapy to 86% (267/310) post-therapy ($p<0.01$).*

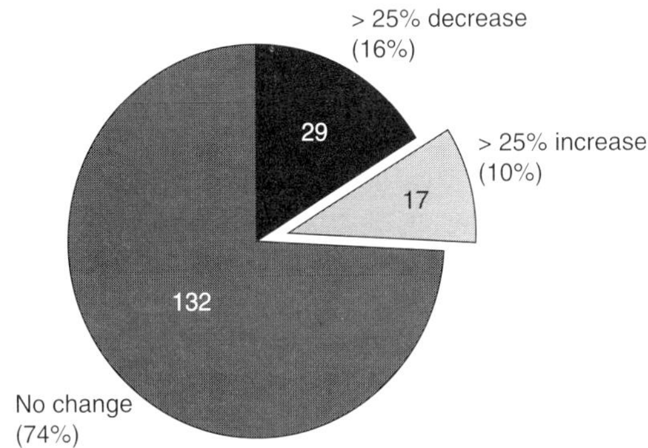

Figure 3.5 *Bladder capacity pressure (BCP) in patients who responded to bladder stimulation with a >20% increase in bladder capacity.*

to pretherapy levels with no further therapy, two patients still have significantly elevated storage pressures and are being followed carefully while continuing further bladder stimulation, and five patients have been lost to follow-up.

Interestingly, further evaluation of the patients who did not respond to bladder stimulation therapy (nonresponders, with a >20% in BC), comparing them to those who did (responders), reveals a significant difference in their pretherapy percent EBC. The nonresponders had a pretherapy percent EBC of 83%, while the responders' pretherapy percent EBC was 65%. In other words, the nonresponders had a bladder capacity which was much closer to normal than the responders. This suggests that bladder stimulation therapy has a greater effect on bladder capacity when the pretherapy capacity is markedly less than normal than when it is close to normal. This also implies that bladder stimulation may be less effective in patients with a large-capacity, atonic bladder.

The final objective of this multi-institutional trial was to address the concern of inconsistent observations between institutions. In an effort to evaluate this, the data set from each institution was separated, to compare the results from patients at CMH (155) with those from the ten other centers (180). Figure 3.6 summarizes the bladder capacity results. One can see that the percentages are similar between the two groups, with CMH having a slightly higher percentage (60% vs. 48%) in the favorable category of patients with a >20% increase in their bladder capacity. This slight variance may be attributed to the fact that the patients at CMH have had longer periods of therapy, compared to the children at the other institutions. Long-term experience has shown that improvements in bladder compliance can still be attained after 1–2 years in some patients with further periodic therapy. There were no other appreciable differences in the results between CMH and the other ten institutions with regard to changes in BC or BCP. These comparisons demonstrate that success with bladder stimulation is not institution specific, and can be duplicated elsewhere.

Several conclusions can be drawn from the results of this multi-institutional trial. First and foremost, it is clear that bladder stimulation is clinically beneficial via its ability to improve bladder compliance through an increase in functional BC and/or decrease in bladder storage pressures. Additionally, these data demonstrate that the favorable results that have been observed at CMH can be achieved in other programs. Lastly, these results reiterate the greater benefit for patients with a small-capacity, poorly compliant bladder.

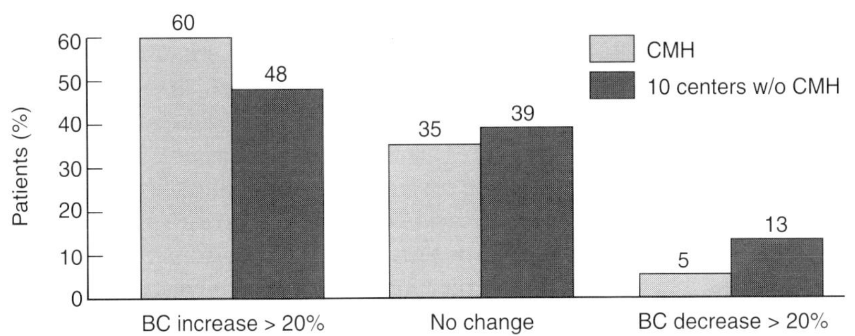

Figure 3.6 *Change in bladder capacity (BC) following bladder stimulation therapy. Comparison of results between Children's Memorial Hospital (CMH) in Chicago and remaining 10 institutions.*

The favorable results of bladder stimulation on bladder compliance prompted the evaluation of whether this therapy is indeed effective in patients with a small, poorly compliant neurogenic bladder, who are otherwise candidates for augmentation cystoplasty. A study was conducted to begin evaluating whether bladder stimulation could be a nonsurgical alternative to bladder augmentation in patients with a severe neurogenic bladder. In this study, the charts of all children treated at CMH with bladder stimulation were reviewed. Those patients with pretreatment 'high-risk' factors defined as: (a) percent expected bladder capacity (PEBC) of 60% or less; and (b) BCP 50 cmH_2O or greater, were identified.[14] Seven patients were found to fit these criteria. Of these seven, three had been referred from outside institutions following a recommendation of bladder augmentation, while the remaining four were from CMH and were likewise being considered for an augmentation procedure should bladder stimulation not be beneficial. All seven patients in this study completed at least two series of bladder stimulation treatments. The mean number of series completed was 4.3 (range = 2–9), and the mean time duration of the treatment course was 1.7 years (range = 1–3 years). Four out of seven patients had substantial increases in PEBC and decreases in BCP. Two out of seven patients responded to therapy with a minimal increase in PEBC but with a notable decrease in BCP. The last patient had an increase in PEBC, but only a modest decrease in BCP. When all seven patients were evaluated as a single group, PEBC increased from an average pretreatment value of 44% to 65% ($p<0.05$) after bladder stimulation therapy. Additionally, BCP improved from an average pretreatment value of 63.9 to 32.3 cmH_2O ($p<0.05$) post-treatment.

All seven patients tolerated the therapy well and there were no noted complications. No patients developed spontaneous voiding following therapy (if they were not voiding pretherapy) and five of seven patients remain on intermittent catheterization. The degree of continence improved in all patients and four of the seven patients are now completely dry. The remaining three out of the seven patients, who still have a mild degree of incontinence, have decreased outlet resistance and will probably require some type of bladder neck procedure if they wish to attain complete dryness. Of greater importance is the fact that these three patients will not require augmentation in addition to a bladder neck procedure, if their improvement from bladder stimulation is maintained. Two out of the seven patients had unilateral grade II–III vesicoureteral reflux, which resolved following therapy. No patients have developed reflux or worsening hydronephrosis during therapy. All seven patients in this series improved their functional bladder capacity and/or improved storage pressures such that surgical intervention has thus far not been undertaken. These results form the basis of primarily treating the high-risk patient with bladder stimulation, rather than with bladder augmentation. Although initial observations seem to indicate that this result is durable, further long-term follow-up and prospective studies will be necessary to determine the long-term efficacy and appropriateness of this therapy in these types of patients.

Case report

ME is a 14-year-old boy with a neurogenic bladder, secondary to myelomeningocele. At the age of 9 he was referred from an outside center to CMH for bladder stimulation therapy. Previous urodynamic studies demonstrated that he had a small noncompliant bladder with a BC of 75–100 cm^3, a BCP of 60–100 cmH_2O, uninhibited contractions, and evidence of an incompetent outlet. Prior management included a regimen of intermittent catheterization (although he did have the ability to void spontaneously) and anticholinergic therapy, which was minimally effective. A bladder augmentation procedure in conjunction with placement of an artificial sphincter was proposed if a trial of bladder stimulation failed.

Over a 3-year period, ME underwent a total of 70 outpatient sessions of bladder stimulation. At the conclusion of therapy, he had a marked increase in bladder capacity (336 cm^3) and reduction in BCP (24 cmH_2O). This improvement was not always apparent on interval urodynamic studies, as seen in Fig. 3.7, which illustrates the 'staircase' pattern in his progress with respect to bladder capacity. Recently, ME returned for a follow-up urodynamic study. His parameters have continued to improve, despite not

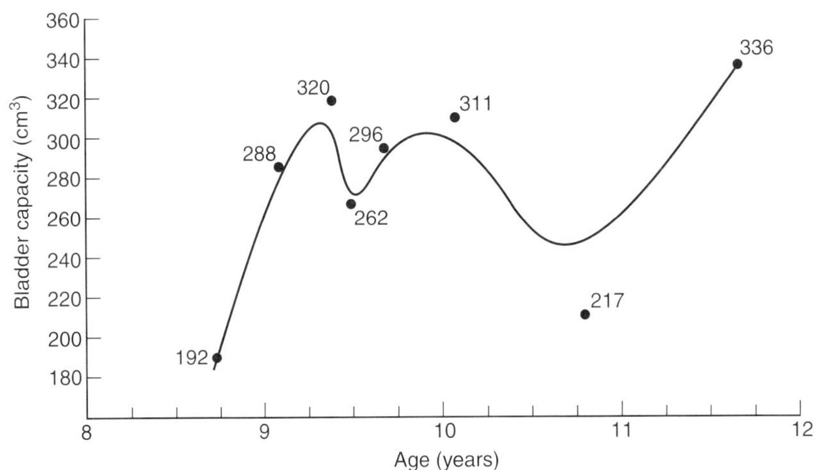

Figure 3.7 *Case report (ME): bladder capacity (BC) measurements during therapy. Note 'staircase'-like pattern: improvement followed by stabilization or diminution, followed by further improvement with persistent therapy.*

having any bladder stimulation treatments for the past 6 years. His BC is currently 500 cm^3 with a BCP of 20 cmH_2O. No uninhibited contractions are present. Clinically, he spontaneously voids to completion and is off anticholinergic medications. He still has some persistent urinary incontinence with increased abdominal pressure, which is probably secondary to a partially incompetent bladder neck.

This case report illustrates several important points regarding bladder stimulation therapy in children with a noncompliant bladder. Most importantly, it demonstrates that bladder stimulation therapy can be successful in some children who are refractory to a program of clean intermittent catheterization and pharmacotherapy, and that this may be a viable alternative to enterocystoplasty. Also, the 'staircase' pattern (i.e., significant improvement, some diminution, followed by further improvement) with respect to his measured bladder capacity is important, since it is seen in the majority of patients receiving bladder stimulation for a noncompliant bladder. Even though primary failure can occur, one must have patience with this therapy and not quickly discontinue treatment if one poor BC measurement is obtained early in the course of treatment. Continued therapy will usually result in renewed improvement in capacity, and further gains will be achieved. Lastly, ME's recent follow-up urodynamic study demonstrates that the improved compliance achieved with this therapy can be durable, and that further growth of the bladder is continued in the absence of continued therapy. Although ME may need an outlet resistance procedure to achieve total dryness, the need for a concurrent bladder augmentation and its associated potential complications has been avoided through the use of bladder stimulation therapy.

Conclusions

Intravesical transurethral bladder stimulation is a valuable diagnostic and rehabilitative procedure that has been found to be successful in initiating sensory-induced detrusor contractions. The ultimate goal in this therapy is to create conscious urinary control. While this goal is indeed achievable in some patients, it has been recognized that the majority of patients are not able to develop complete conscious control of their lower urinary tract after undergoing this therapy. Nevertheless, patients undergoing this therapy still clearly benefit in other ways. The combination of an increase in sensation of bladder filling, an increase in bladder capacity, and maintenance of safe bladder storage pressures is seen in a majority of patients. This translates clinically into improved urinary continence, increased awareness of the need to catheterize, increased time interval between catheterizations, and the need for less medication. As suggested by some, even greater benefit and improvement may be gained if bladder stimulation is initiated in the first year of life to avoid the development of irreversible fibrotic changes in the bladder. Although further experience is needed, it now appears that bladder stimulation therapy may be most appropriate for patients with a small-capacity and poorly compliant bladder. Major benefits of therapy are an improvement in bladder compliance through an increase in bladder capacity and/or lowering of bladder storage pressures. This improvement may be enough to obviate the need for a bladder augmentation procedure in some patients. Despite initial encouraging results, the recommendation that bladder stimulation should replace augmentation in the majority of patients with a small, noncompliant, neurogenic bladder cannot be made at this time. Further experience and long-term follow-up are needed. One must also remember that families and patients have to be extremely motivated and reliable for bladder stimulation to be successful, since this therapy is labor intensive and requires a significant time commitment. However, it is reasonable to at least consider this therapy as an alternative to bladder augmentation in selected patients. When properly administered, bladder stimulation is safe, has little-to-no associated complications, and can be very successful.

SACRAL RHIZOTOMY

As with bladder stimulation, sacral rhizotomy also represents a possible alternative to bladder augmentation in the management of children with a neurogenic bladder. Alteration of urinary tract dynamics by surgical interruption of the nervous supply is a concept which has been attempted in the past in various forms. In general, these procedures have produced less than desirable results. This may in large part be due to the nonselective nature of the rhizotomy and to the resultant effects on pelvic floor innervation and function.[15,16] The recent introduction of selective sacral rhizotomy to manage lower extremity spasticity in children with cerebral palsy[17] and myelomeningocele[18] has rekindled interest in treating neurologic dysfunction of the urinary tract with surgical alteration of the innervation of the bladder. This interest was further heightened by the observation that urinary tract dynamics improved in those children who had selective sacral rhizotomies performed primarily for limb spasticity. The presumed mechanism of action of this therapy is to interrupt the sensory nerves involved in the spinal afferent loop and thus abolish reflex bladder contractions, while maintaining motor innervation of the detrusor and pelvic floor. With improved neurosurgical techniques, it is clear from preliminary results that this can be accomplished in both children and adults, and that selective sacral rhizotomy is a viable alternative for the primary management of the neurogenic bladder in patients who are not responsive to more conventional medical management.

Selective sacral rhizotomy technique

Patients are selected for sacral rhizotomy based upon the following criteria: (a) continued deterioration of urodynamic parameters and/or upper urinary tract dilation despite aggressive medical management (including clear intermittent catheterization and pharmacotherapy); or (b) severe lower extremity spasticity in conjunction with a high-pressure neurogenic bladder. Following the induction of anesthesia, a Foley catheter is placed in the bladder for the purpose of monitoring bladder pressure during the procedure while the patient is in the supine position. Perineal electromyography activity is also monitored continuously. Initial experience with pacing wires placed in the detrusor wall has not proved them to be beneficial, and they are no longer routinely used.[19] The patient is then placed in the prone position and sacral spinal nerves are exposed, intradurally, at the point of exit from the spinal cord.

Once exposure of the nerve roots is complete, the motor roots are verified electrophysiologically by their unique stimulation pattern and separated from the sensory roots. Each sensory root is then further divided into its component rootlets (usually three to 15 in number) and each rootlet is stimulated sequentially. Individual sensory rootlets are stimulated at 1 and 50 Hz. Normal sensory roots have a brisk single stimulus threshold much higher than motor rootlets, with rapid relaxation of muscular contraction. Further specific electrophysiologic stimulation is performed as previously described.[15,19]

Detrusor activity and bladder pressure are monitored continuously during rootlet stimulation. Rootlets which produce a definitive detrusor contraction and no simultaneous contraction of the external sphincter are sectioned with microscissors without electrocoagulation. If no bladder contraction is observed but a significant increase in tone of the muscle wall is noted, these rootlets are also cut. If sphincter activity is present along with detrusor activity, further dissection of the rootlet is undertaken to isolate the segment responsible for the detrusor response. Following completion of selective dorsal nerve transections, the procedure is terminated. Postoperative urodynamic and radiographic evaluation at 6 weeks and 6 months is routinely performed.

Results

Since 1987, 11 patients have been treated at CMH with selective sacral rhizotomy as a method of management of their urinary tract. All patients were refractory to medical management. The level of the lesion varied, including lumbar in five, thoracic in two, sacral in two, and sacral agenesis in two. Schneidau *et al.* (1995)[19] recently reported on the long-term follow-up (12–49 months) of these patients. Overall, there was an 84% increase in bladder volume. More importantly, uninhibited contractions were abolished in all patients. Bladder volume at a pressure of 40 cmH_2O increased 93% from preoperative levels. Pelvic floor innervation does not appear to be injured by selective rhizotomy since the leak-point pressure was not significantly altered in these patients following surgery. Clinically, no patient experienced worsening incontinence secondary to injury to sphincter innervation.

Again, as with bladder stimulation, it appears that early intervention, as opposed to later, may be most beneficial and advantageous for the patient with a neurogenic bladder. In the above-described study by Shneidau *et al.*,[19] not all 11 patients had a marked improvement in bladder capacity and bladder compliance. If the data are further stratified to separate younger from older patients (age greater than 9 years old), a much more favorable response is observed in the younger children. In fact, a 169% increase in bladder capacity is seen in the younger group. This suggests that younger children, whose bladders are presumably less fibrotic, respond more favorably than older children. The advantage of early institution of therapy is further supported by experience with selective sacral rhizotomy in adult spinal cord-injured patients. In 1992, Gasparini *et al.*[16] reported on the use of this technique in 17 patients with spinal cord injuries, ranging in age from 26 to 53 years. Interestingly, patients with an injury of less than 5 years' duration had a more predictable and positive outcome with regard to an increase in bladder capacity, than those patients with injuries present for longer than 5 years. Collectively, these data suggest that prolonged dysfunction of the detrusor wall may result in irreversible fibrotic changes which will be less responsive to selective sacral rhizotomy. Despite this, significant improvement can still be achieved in some patients with long-standing injuries. As with bladder stimulation, additional experience is needed to identify additional prognostic indicators for success in order to better select appropriate patients who will have a positive response to therapy.

SUMMARY

We are a long way from a thorough understanding of the neurourological interrelationships in the bladder. The intricate relationship that exists between the nervous system and the bladder is not static, and may change with time in both the normal and the pathological bladder. In patients with spinal dysraphism and neurogenic bladder disease, the degree of plasticity of the neuromotor unit in the bladder wall may remain favorable and receptive to therapeutic intervention for many years. It is clear that nerves can be altered and 'rescued' during these favorable years with either intravesical bladder stimulation or selective sacral rhizotomy, to achieve a more clinically manageable bladder. However, additional creativity in thought regarding the modulation of the neuromuscular unit in the bladder is definitely needed to improve on our current therapy. Also, there is a tremendous need for additional basic scientific knowledge of the pathophysiology and mechanism of action of these therapies. Answers to important questions regarding changes in bladder histology, cellular structure, and bladder wall receptors following therapy are still lacking. It is to be hoped that further advances in knowledge will result in new and improved treatment modalities which will enable us to alter the abnormal messages from an impaired nervous system and bladder, leading to functional improvement in bladder wall dynamics. Although additional work is needed, clinical experience has clearly shown that both intravesical bladder stimulation and selective sacral rhizotomy are of benefit to selected patients with a neurogenic bladder.

REFERENCES

1. Katona, F. and Berenyi, M. (1975) Intravesical transurethral electrotherapy in meningomyelocele patients. *Acta Paediatrica Hungarica,* **16,** 363.
2. Madersbacher, H., Pauer, W. and Reiner, E. (1982) Rehabilitation of micturition by transurethral electrostimulation of the bladder in patients with incomplete spinal cord lesions. *Paraplegia,* **20,** 191–5.
3. Kaplan, W.E. and Richards, I. (1986) Intravesical transurethral electrotherapy for the neurogenic bladder. *Journal of Urology,* **136,** 243–6.
4. Kaplan, W.E. and Richards, I. (1988) Intravesical bladder stimulation in myelodysplasia. *Journal of Urology,* **140,** 1282–4.
5. Ebner, A., Jiang, C. and Lindstrom, S. (1992) Intravesical electrical stimulation – an experimental analysis of the mechanism of action. *Journal of Urology,* **148,** 920–4.
6. Kaplan, W.E., Richards, T.W. and Richards, I. (1989) Intravesical transurethral bladder stimulation to increase bladder capacity. *Journal of Urology,* **142,** 600–2.
7. Kaplan, W.E. (1994) Alternative to enterocystoplasty: bladder stimulation. *Problems in Urology,* **8** (3), 410–15.
8. Berger, R.M., Maizels, M., Morgan, G.C. *et al.* (1983) Bladder capacity (ounces) equals age (years) plus two predicts normal bladder capacity and aids in diagnosis of abnormal voiding patterns. *Journal of Urology,* **129,** 347–9.
9. Boone, T.B., Roehrborn C.G. and Hurt, G. (1992) Transurethral intravesical electrotherapy for neurogenic bladder dysfunction in children with myelodysplasia: a prospective randomised clinical trial. *Journal of Urology,* **148,** 550–4.
10. Lyne, C.J. and Bellinger, M.F. (1993) Early experience with transurethral electrical bladder stimulation. *Journal of Urology,* **150,** 697–9.
11. Decter, R.M., Snyder, P. and Laudermilch, C. (1994) Transurethral electrical bladder stimulation: a follow up report. *Journal of Urology,* **152,** 812–14.
12. Cheng, E.Y., Richards, I., Balcom, A. *et al.* (1996) Bladder stimulation therapy improves bladder compliance: results from multi-institutional trial. *Journal of Urology,* **156,** 761–4.
13. McGuire, E.J., Woodside, J.R., Bordern, T.A. *et al.* (1981) Prognostic value of urodynamics testing in myelodysplastic patients. *Journal of Urology,* **126,** 205–9.
14. Cheng, E.Y., Richards, I. and Kaplan, W.E. (1996) Use of bladder stimulation in high risk patients. *Journal of Urology,* **156,** 749–52.
15. Franco, I., Storrs, B., Firlit, C.F. *et al.* (1992) Selective sacral rhizotomy in children with high pressure neurogenic bladders: preliminary results. *Journal of Urology,* **148,** 648–50.
16. Gasparini, M.E., Schmidt, R.A. and Tanagho, E.A. (1992) Selective sacral rhizotomy in the management of the reflex neuropathic bladder: a report on 17 patients with long-term follow-up. *Journal of Urology,* **148,** 1207–10.
17. Peacock, W.J., Arens, L.J. and Berman, B. (1987) Cerebral palsy spasticity. Selective posterior rhizotomy. *Pediatric Neuroscience,* **13,** 61–2.
18. Storrs, B.B. (1987) Selective posterior rhizotomy for treatment of progressive spasticity in patients with myelomeningocele. Preliminary report. *Pediatric Neuroscience,* **13,** 135–7.
19. Schneidau, T., Franco, I., Zebold, K. *et al.* (1995) Selective sacral rhizotomy for the management of neurogenic bladders in spina bifida patients: long-term follow-up. *Journal of Urology,* **154,** 766–8.

4

Supratrigonal bladder transection

PADDY DEWAN

INTRODUCTION

The neuropathic bladder can usually be managed conservatively, using anticholinergic medication and intermittent catheterization, or with the addition of techniques suggested in Chapters 2 and 3. In a small number of cases, augmentation is indicated in those patients with a small-capacity, high-pressure bladder, to achieve continence and prevent renal damage. In recent years, there have been many studies aimed at developing new methods of bladder enlargement, particularly in an attempt to achieve a urothelial-lined reservoir.[1–10] The literature reports bladder augmentation studies in a number of different species, including the rat, rabbit, dog, calf, pig, and sheep, but only in Mau's study[11] was there an attempt to create a neuropathic bladder prior to the augmentation procedure. However, Mau's method produced a more widespread neurological insult. Sethia *et al.*[12] produced unstable contractions in the minipig bladder by a circumferential supratrigonal incision. Gonzalez *et al.* produced non-neurogenic contractions of the canine bladder by removal of its serosal surface,[2] Staskin *et al.*[13] found a decrease in the bladder capacity following bladder transection in the dog, Choudhury and Mittra[14] created a bladder with normal, but altered function, by division of the posterior portion of the supratrigonal bladder in the dog. This resulted in a higher volume, lower pressure bladder with essentially normal contractions.

To date, animal studies of new techniques of bladder augmentation are necessarily based on the normal urinary bladder because a suitable animal model for the human neuropathic bladder has not yet been established. Ideally, such augmentation procedures should be tested in an animal model with a contracted, high-pressure bladder similar to that seen in the spina bifida child, in whom bladder augmentation is usually performed. Therefore, as previous animal studies had reported the development of features of a neurogenic bladder by a supratrigonal bladder transection, a series of sheep were studied to assess the validity of the model and the effect of bladder dynamics, during which a suprapubic urodynamic catheter was used.[15]

Paradoxically, the median volume for a group of ten sheep with supratrigonal bladder transection increased significantly from 86 ml at 6 months to 245 ml at 12 months. At 12 months, the median volume for the control group was 165 ml. There was no significant difference between the transection and control groups at 12 months (p=0.18). One of the

Table 4.1 *Bladder volumes of the study group animals immediately before the supratrigonal transection, at 6 months of age (Preop.) and again 6 months later, when the sheep were 12 months old (Postop.)*

Sheep no.	Study group Volume at leak pressure (ml)	
	Preop.	Postop.
1	109	199
2	132	60
3	88	211
4	84	339
6	61	222
7	36	276
8	58	427
9	123	314
10	107	268
Median	86	245

transected animals had a decreased bladder volume which was thought to be due to ischemia at the time of the transection. All other animals had an increase in bladder volume and no unstable contractions were seen in any of the urodynamic studies. The results of this study are given in Tables 4.1 and 4.2 (see also Figs. 4.1 and 4.2).

Therefore, supratrigonal bladder transection in the sheep does not appear to produce an adequate model for the human neurogenic bladder. A review of the literature highlights the variable outcome of the bladder transection technique both in animal studies and in the clinical application of the technique.

Table 4.2 *Bladder volumes of six control group animals aged 12–14 months*

Sheep no.	Study group Volume at leak pressure (ml) 12 months
1	143
2	169
3	244
4	105
5	160
6	304
Median	165

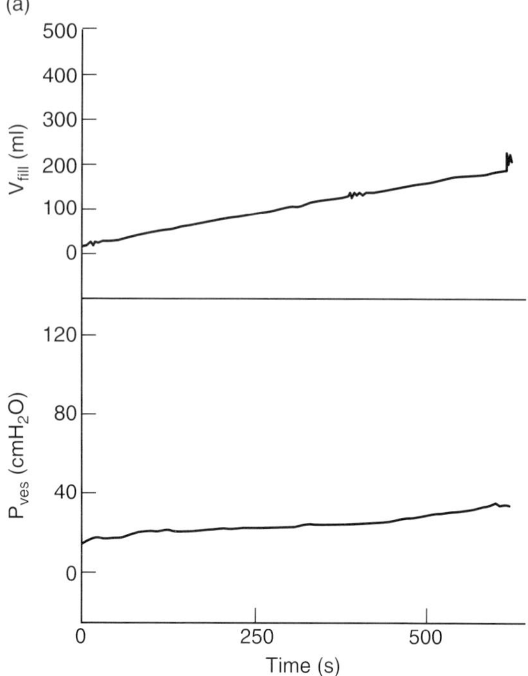

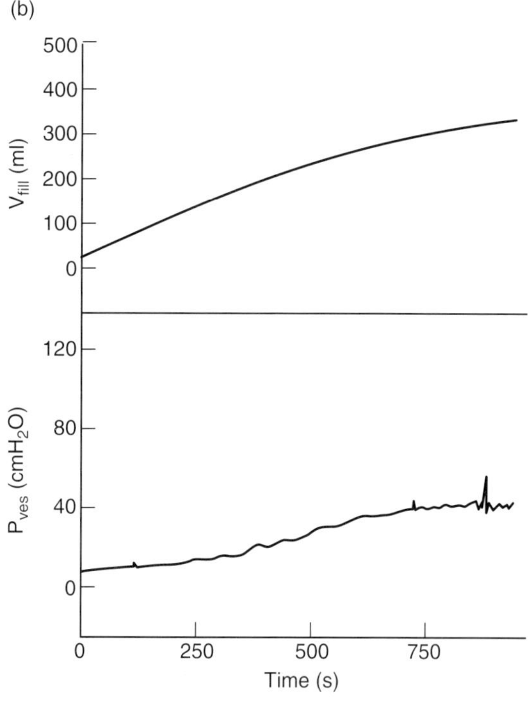

Figure 4.1 *A urodynamic study (a) before and (b) 6 months after the transection. P_{ves}, vesical pressure; V_{fill}, fill volume.*

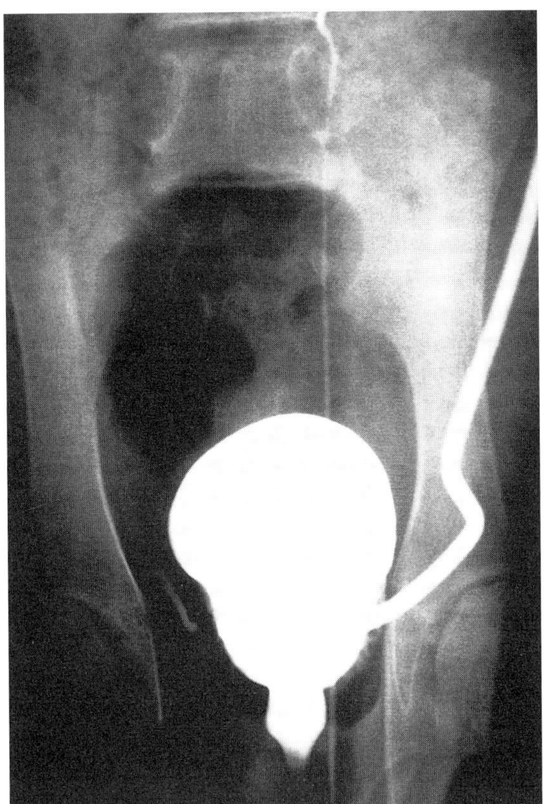

Figure 4.2 *A cystogram 10 days after the supratrigonal incision.*

ANIMAL STUDIES

The above study has shown that, in the sheep, supratrigonal transection produces neither unstable bladder contractions nor a significant difference in bladder volume. These results contrast with the findings of Sethia *et al.*[12] who used a supratrigonal transection of the minipig bladder and found bladder instability but no change in compliance at 3 weeks in all of their eight minipigs. They did not find any increase in the density of the cholinergic nerve fibres, but recorded increased sensitivity to carbachol, potassium and acetylcholine in the muscular strips from the transected bladders versus the control bladders. Staskin *et al.*[13] found supersensitivity to bethanocol following bladder transection, but with a reputed increase in the density of cholinergic receptors in dogs and rabbits. Unlike our findings, they found a decrease in the bladder capacity. This may relate to the relatively early sacrifice of their animals at 120 days.[13]

Choudhury and Mittra[14] also found altered bladder function in a dog model after posterior supratrigonal transection–denervation of the bladder; their results, however, differ from those of Sethia *et al.* in that they produced an enlarged bladder at 4 weeks with no unstable contractions.[14] Interestingly, Sibley[16] found changes in the obstructed pig bladder consistent with partial denervation, with increased sensitivity to acetylcholine and potassium, but decreased responsiveness to nerve stimulation of muscle strips. These changes are similar to those found by others after surgical denervation of the rat, cat, and dog bladder.

Overall, the animal studies have had varied results, which may relate to species differences and subtle differences in the operative techniques. The conclusion must be that the highly predictable development of a neurogenic bladder that would fit with the currently available literature on the clinical use of bladder transection has not been possible.

CLINICAL USE OF BLADDER TRANSECTION

While supratrigonal bladder transection has been used in the normal animal bladder in an attempt to create the features of a neuropathic bladder, it has also been reported as a surgical method for denervation of the bladder of patients with unstable contractions.

Essenhigh and Yeates[17] reported the use of open supratrigonal transection in 15 adults with a clinical history suggestive of bladder instability but a stable bladder under anaesthetic. Their cases were selected without detailed cystometric investigation and seven were followed for less than 1 year, and 13 for less than 2 years. Improvement in day-time symptoms was reported as 'excellent' or 'very good' in 11 patients, 'good' in three, and 'improved' in one. Essenhigh[18] was subsequently involved in a report of 50 patients undergoing an endoscopic bladder transection, in whom the procedure was deemed successful in only 16%. Bladder instability was demonstrated in all patients before operation and in 93% postoperatively. Lucas and Thomas[19] had similarly poor results using an endoscopic approach, whereas Parsons *et al.*[20] had better results, with an excellent outcome in 57% of 30 patients and no change in 18%; they recommended further use of the technique.

In contrast to the animal study results, Turner-Warwick and Ashken[21] have described 'supratrigonal denervation' for a hypersensitive bladder. They used the 'cystoplasty' on a 58-year-old woman with reduction of her bladder spasms. Gibbon *et al.*[22] performed a supratrigonal transection in seven patients with bladder instability and a normal bladder capacity, curing two completely and improving the other five. The bladder instability status of the group, however, was not discussed in detail and Gibbon *et al.* did not divide the inferior vesical vessels, as had been done by Turner-Warwick and Ashken.[21]

Janknegt *et al.*[23] used the open technique of Essenhigh and Yeates, producing improvement in two patients and good results in five. Bladder instability was present in one patient with a good result and in one with improvement. Six patients had night wetting only and all of these had a stable bladder preoperatively and postoperatively. The second of two studies published in 1995 suggested that the results in 12 patients in whom an open operation left a bridge of tissue above the left ureteric orifice were encouraging, but only three were cured, seven were improved, and two had not changed.

Overall, it would seem that supratrigonal transection has poorly predictable results both clinically and in animal models, thus having limited application in the clinical management of bladder dysfunction in humans and the formation of a neurogenic bladder model in animals.

REFERENCES

1. Dewan, P.A. and Byard, R.W. (1993) Autoaugmentation gastrocystoplasty in a sheep model. *British Journal of Urology,* **72**, 56–9.
2. Gonzalez, R., Buson, H., Reid, C. *et al.* (1995) Seromuscular colocystoplasty lined with urothelium: experience with 16 patients. *Urology,* **45**, 124–9.
3. Dewan, P.A. and Stefanek, W. (1994) Autoaugmentation colocystoplasty: a case report. *Pediatric Surgery International,* **9**, 526–8.
4. Dewan, P.A., Lorenz, C., Stefanek, W. *et al.* (1994) Urothelial lined colocystoplasty in a sheep model. *European Urology,* **26,** 240–6.
5. Robinson, R.G., Delahunt, B. and Pringle, KC. (1994) Autoaugmentation gastrocystoplasty. *Journal of Urology,* **151**, Suppl., 500A (abstract).
6. Horowitz, M., Mitchell, M.E. and Nguyen, D.H. (1994) The DAWG procedure, gastrocystoplasty made better. *Journal of Urology*; **151**, Suppl., 503A (abstract).
7. Dewan, P.A., Stefanek, W., Lorenz, C. *et al.* (1995) Autoaugmentation gastrocystoplasty and demucosalised gastrocystoplasty in a sheep model. *Urology,* **45**, 291–5.
8. Dewan, P.A. and Stefanek, W. (1994) Autoaugmentation gastrocystoplasty: early clinical results. *British Journal of Urology,* **74,** 460–4.
9. Lima, S.V.C., Araujo, L.A.P., Vilar, F.O. *et al.* (1995) Nonsecretory sigmoid cystoplasty: experimental and clinical results. *Journal of Urology,* **153**, 1651–4.
10. Buson, H., Manivel, J.C., Dayanç, M. *et al.* (1994) Seromuscular colocystoplasty lined with urothelium (SCLU): experimental study. *Urology,* **44,** 743–8.
11. Mau, H. (1980) Die neurogene Blase – tierexperimentelle Untersuchungen zur Restauration der Blasenfunktion. Habilitationsschrift, Humboldt-Universität zu Berlin, 1–300.
12. Sethia, K.K., Brading, A.F. and Smith, J.C. (1990) An animal model of non-obstructive bladder instability. *Journal of Urology,* **143**, 1243–6.
13. Staskin, D.R., Parsons, K.F. and Levin, R.M. (1981) Bladder transection – a functional, neurophysiological, neuropharmacological and neuroanatomical study. *British Journal of Urology,* **53**, 552–7.
14. Choudhury, A. and Mittra, S. (1980) Transection denervation of the urinary bladder: an experimental study. *British Journal of Urology,* **52**, 193–5.

15. Dewan, P.A. (1995) A double lumen suprapubic urodynamic catheter. *Australian and New Zealand Journal of Surgery,* **65**, 672–3.
16. Sibley, G.N.A. (1987) The physiological response of the detrusor muscle to experimental bladder outflow obstruction. *British Journal of Urology,* **60**, 332–6.
17. Essenhigh, D.M. and Yeates, W.K. (1973) Transection of the bladder with particular reference to enuresis. *British Journal of Urology,* **45**, 299–305.
18. Hasan, S.T., Robson, W.A., Ramsden, P.D. *et al.* (1995) Outcome of endoscopic bladder transection. *British Journal of Urology,* **75**, 592–6.
19. Lucas, M.G. and Thomas, D.G. (1987) Endoscopic bladder transection for detrusor instability. *British Journal of Urology,* **59**, 526–8.
20. Parsons, K.F., Machin, D.G., Woolfenden, K.A. *et al.*, (1984) Endoscopic bladder transection. *British Journal of Urology,* **56**, 625–8.
21. Turner-Warwick, R.T. and Ashken, M.H. (1967) The functional results of partial, subtotal and total cystoplasty with special reference to ureterocaecoplasty, selective sphincterotomy and cystocystoplasty. *British Journal of Urology,* **39**, 3–12.
22. Gibbon, N.O.K., Jameson, R.M., Heal, M.R. *et al,* (1973) Transection of the bladder for adult enuresis and allied conditions. *British Journal of Urology,* **45**, 306–9.
23. Janknegt, R.A., Moonen, W.A. and Schreinemachers, L.M.H. (1979) Transection of the bladder as a method of treatment in adult enuresis noctura. *British Journal of Urology,* **51**, 275–7.

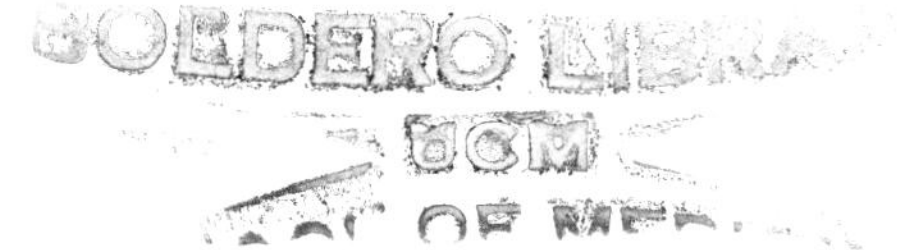

5

Small and large bowel enterocystoplasty

MICHAEL C CARR

INTRODUCTION

The use of bowel in total lower urinary tract reconstruction had its practical genesis in Gilchrist's[1] procedure for 'a substitution bladder and urethra.' The cecum and ascending colon, along with a segment of terminal ileum, were used. The ureters were reimplanted submucosally and the ileal urethra was brought out in the right lower quadrant of the abdomen. Continence was excellent postoperatively, although catheterization was, at times, difficult. Gilchrist recommended fixing the 'new urethra' in a straight line from the abdomen to the ileocecal valve without angulation. He also recommended catheterization often enough to prevent overfilling (intermittent catheterization). At the same time, Bricker[2] proposed the construction of an ileal conduit, comprised of a uretero-enterocutaneous anastomosis. This technique gained wider acceptance as a means for urinary diversion for many adult and pediatric patients with complex urologic problems. The long-term sequelae of ileal conduit urinary diversion were appreciated 20 years later, as upper tract deterioration was increasingly being detected. During this era, augmentation cystoplasty was reserved only for patients with an ability to empty. In fact, it was the popular notion that augmentation in neurogenic bladder patients was contraindicated. This concept rapidly changed with the popularization of clean intermittent catheterization (CIC) by Lapides[3] in the early 1970s. These events stimulated renewed interest in urinary undiversion, combining enterocystoplasty to improve bladder compliance and provide the means for management of urinary continence following undiversion even in those patients with neuropathic bladder.[4–7]

Enterocystoplasties have been routinely performed for the past 15–20 years and the complications associated with these procedures have come to our attention. Bladder perforation, infection, stone formation, metabolic abnormality, mucus production, and the threat of malignant transformation have led to newer methods of bladder augmentation. These topics are discussed in Chapters 6 and 7.

PATIENT EVALUATION/PRINCIPLES OF MANAGEMENT

After general acceptance of CIC, bladder augmentation was applied not only to patients with interstitial cystitis, 'defunctionalized bladders,' radiation cystitis, tuberculosis, and chemical cystitis,[8,9] but also to neurogenic bladder patients. The majority of pediatric patients requiring augmentation have a 'neurogenic bladder' secondary to myelodysplasia, but a second category of patients includes those with congenital malformations such as exstrophy, cloacal malformation, and posterior urethral obstruction. The emphasis in this era of molecular biology, in which we are beginning to gain an appreciation for how the bladder develops and maintains itself, is to make every effort to prevent the need for bladder augmentation.

A thorough history will include details of a patient's previous medical management. In the evaluation of a wet patient, what is the current management of the bladder? Has the pharmacologic management been optimized? Is the patient adhering to a consistent program of catheterization and how compliant is the patient? Does the patient have any difficulties with catheterization? What prior surgery has been performed on the bladder neck? Have any complications occurred, such as erosion of an artificial urinary sphincter or perforation of an augmented bladder? Has prior ureteroneocystostomy been performed? Is an appendix present? A history of nephrolithiasis, impaired renal function, hypertension and polyuria needs to be evaluated and clearly assessed prior to augmentation. Perhaps more significant, however, are 'nonmedical' factors such as the patient's motivation, intellectual function, manual dexterity, and family support systems, which will all have a major influence on the ultimate success of the procedure.

The physical examination must include a thorough assessment of the patient's overall condition and body habitus. The upper and lower extremity neurologic status should be carefully assessed. Further considerations include tone of the anal sphincter and perineal musculature. The abdomen needs to be evaluated for potential placement of the catheterizable stoma. Further considerations include whether the patient is ambulatory or wheelchair dependent. Ambulation with crutches can place significant demands on the continence mechanism. A heavy-set child in a wheelchair may not be able to activate an artificial urinary sphincter or easily catheterize using her or his urethra, but could manage very well with a continent catheterizable stoma to the umbilicus. Most importantly, in the assessment of the patient should include the realistic consideration of the ability to perform self-catheterization. Without confidence that CIC can be carried out regularly and dependably, no consideration for augmentation can be made. Furthermore, the overall bowel continence and success of the bowel program should be assessed as well. The construction of a catheterizable channel to the cecum (ACE, antegrade continence enema) could be accomplished and should be considered at the time of bladder augmentation.[10,11]

The social pressures to be dry are certainly great. Parents are eager for their children to be free of diapers. The alternative is a program of CIC, which may already be well established. It is imperative that this is well accepted and already in place before an augmentation procedure is embarked upon. Children with a sensate urethra are much less likely to adhere to a catheterization program. In these cases a continent catheterizable stoma (Mitrofanoff) should be considered.[12]

As children enter adolescence, their motivation to continue with the catheterization program may decline. This, in part, can be due to their need to be normal, so that noncompliance becomes a form of denial. This can become a critical issue, particularly if the leak-point pressure is high, such as exists with an artificial urinary sphincter or closed bladder neck. The patient at greatest risk of bladder perforation is the one who has been most 'successful' with an augmentation, being completely dry with no sensation of bladder fullness.

It becomes very important to assess the social situation and the support structures that are available to families. The ability of the family to deal with surgical complications and aberrations also needs careful assessment. This can obviously not be accomplished in a single visit with the surgeon. The input of an experienced urologic nurse and even a social worker may help identify potential problems before surgery. The establishment of this relationship with the urologic team and with local support systems is necessary preoperatively, particularly if patients live a long distance away from the medical center.

Despite all the advance preparations, the patient's and the family's response to surgery or to the surgical complications cannot always be predicted. The surgical team (surgeon and support staff) must be both willing and able to provide the support needed during the stressful and difficult times.

RADIOGRAPHIC AND URODYNAMIC CONSIDERATIONS

The mainstay of understanding the function of the lower urinary tract is the urodynamic evaluation. In many situations, several studies have been done over the years to assess this function. It is equally important to assess the health of the upper urinary tracts. In children, routine ultrasonography has replaced the excretory urogram in this regard. The size of the kidneys, adequacy of renal parenchyma, and dilation of the collecting system are easily noted. Nuclear renography is helpful in determining differential function or evidence of parenchymal scarring (DMSA scan) while diuretic renography (MAG-3 Lasix renogram) provides additional information about washout of radiotracer. This information may be somewhat difficult to interpret with significant dilation of collecting system and ureters or poorly functioning kidneys.

Urodynamic studies are critical for surgical decision-making and ideally are performed with video fluoroscopy. Use of electromyography in conjunction with the cystometrogram can provide information about external urinary sphincter coordination and function as well.

A number of factors are defined with the urodynamic evaluation (Table 5.1).

Several formulas have been proposed for calculating bladder capacity: e.g., under 2 years of age, weight (kg) × 7 = capacity (ml); over 2 years of age, age (years) + 2 = capacity (fl oz). This latter formula would be applicable until a child reaches age 12 or so, when the expected bladder capacity is approximately 400 mL.

Table 5.1 *Parameters assessed with video urodynamics*

1. Obstruction of the upper tracts – either by a mechanical blockage or by functionally inadequate drainage or emptying.
2. Ureteral length and degree of dilation.
3. Bladder capacity.
4. Bladder compliance.
5. Presence of vesicoureteral reflux.
6. Degree of bladder emptying by Valsalva or detrusor contraction.
7. Coordination of bladder neck and external sphincter with voiding.
8. Urethral patency.
9. Leak-point pressure or degree of outflow resistance.[13]

Compliance simply quantitates the ability of a bladder to maintain a given pressure at a given volume. A ratio of V (change in volume)/P (change in pressure) at capacity can provide a numerical estimation of compliance. A compliance that is greater than 10–20 ml/cmH_2O is considered relatively normal, whereas a compliance less than 10 ml/cmH_2O is worrisome and may mean that bladder augmentation is necessary. Several issues must be addressed, though. The compliance is only useful in those patients who demonstrate a relatively constant upward slope to the tonus limb of the cystometrogram curve. Detrusor hyperreflexia or uninhibited bladder contractions can be present, but are not accounted for with compliance measurements. The ratio cannot differentiate between a small fibrotic bladder and a small bladder with the potential to 'stretch up' if it has been defunctionalized.

A concept that may be useful in determining whether augmentation is necessary is defining the Red Zone. The Red Zone is the bladder volume beyond which the bladder pressure exceeds 30 cmH_2O. Prior work has shown the detrimental effects of sustained pressures of greater than 40 cmH_2O.[14] Volume thus becomes the key factor in this situation. Bladder capacity is often quite arbitrarily defined, since this volume can vary greatly between a child who voids volitionally versus a child who is dependent on catheterization for emptying. For example, a 6-year-old myelomeningocele child who has a bladder compliance of 7 ml/cmH_2O would enter the Red Zone (>30 cmH_2O) at a volume of 210 ml. This assumes a rather constant upward slope to the tonus limb. The child's predicted bladder capacity is 240 ml and if he is being catheterized at his capacity, then his bladder is in the Red Zone for 13% of the time. This same child at age 10 with an identical compliance could be in much worse shape. The predicted bladder capacity should be 360 ml and if he catheterizes at his 'capacity,' he could be spending 42% of his time in the Red Zone. To protect his upper tracts, he would potentially need to increase the frequency of his catheterizations, decrease overall urine output, or improve overall compliance.

Augmentation of the bladder using detubularized or reconfigured ileum often results in excellent compliance (30–40 ml/cmH_2O). Augmentation with stomach usually yields a compliance in the normal range of 10–20 ml/cmH_2O. In our experience, bladder augmentation with a colonic patch results in a compliance intermediate between that of ileum and gastric tissue, but is very dependent on the length of the segment taken. Stomach and small bowel seem to stretch up with time.

Preoperative urinalysis and urine culture 1 week before the scheduled procedure will identify infected patients and allow for adequate treatment. Preoperatively, broad-spectrum intravenous antibiotics are routine and preoperative bowel preparation with GoLytely can be carried out in the hospital the day before surgery, or a regimen of clear liquids beginning 2 days before surgery can be initiated. Magnesium citrate, which seems to be more palatable than GoLytely, is given 2 days before and again the day prior to surgery. This would allow the bowel preparation to be performed at home so that the patient can be admitted on the day of surgery.

Increasingly, bladder augmentation is being combined with the Mitrofanoff procedure creating a catheterizable channel that is brought to the umbilicus. For patients with a sensate urethra (exstrophy patients and non-neurogenic, neurogenic bladder patients), this procedure is critical so that catheterizations can be performed. Patients with a neurogenic bladder often prefer using the Mitrofanoff because it makes catheterization much easier and certainly facilitates patient compliance in the long term.[15]

PREOPERATIVE WORK-UP

The preoperative assessment is the most important factor before embarking upon an enterocystoplasty. Proper patient evaluation and selection optimize the potential for success. The patient and family must be committed to the preoperative therapy or else one risks a technical success but surgical failure.

Families are counseled to anticipate that their child will need intermittent catheterization following the augmentation procedure. Many children are already on a catheterization program, but the need to comply becomes even more critical following enterocystoplasty. Only after the patient proves that catheterization is no longer necessary can it be stopped, and this certainly becomes the exception rather than the rule. There are, therefore, three aspects of patient selection and evaluation: (a) evaluation of the anatomy, (b) evaluation of the physiology, and (c) evaluation of patient motivation and support systems. All are important, but assessment of good patient motivation is essential.

BLADDER AUGMENTATION: SURGICAL TECHNIQUE

Once the decision has been made to enlarge the bladder, the next step is to choose a surgical strategy. Although a general plan must be established prior to surgery, specific decisions, such as type of bowel or reimplant, must be made at the time of surgery. Multiple options must be available, and the surgeon cannot be locked into a specific plan. Flexibility to do whatever is required at the time of the procedure serves the patient best.

Important factors to be considered in choosing an enteric segment include availability, absence of disease, sufficient pedicle or mesenteric length. Presence of an appendix is important when considering a Mitrofanoff or ACE procedure. An increased incidence of spontaneous perforation in colocystoplasties or enterocystoplasties should make one equally wary of the choice of bowel.[16,17]

Choices of tissue to improve compliance and increase capacity include ileum, ileocecum or

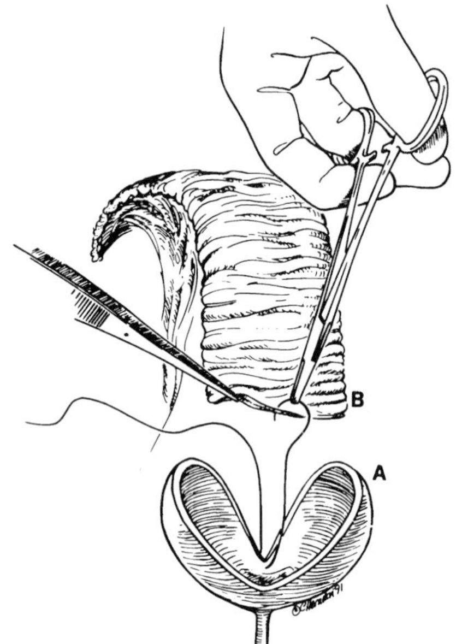

Figure 5.1 *'Clam shell' augmentation cystoplasty. The bladder (A) is split widely from bladder neck anteriorly, almost to the trigone posteriorly. A large patch of ileum (B), opened along its antimesenteric border, is sutured into place. Reproduced with permission from Mitchell, M. and Burns, M.W. (1992)* Urinary Undiversion and Augmentation Cystoplasty. *Philadelphia, W.B. Saunders, Co.*

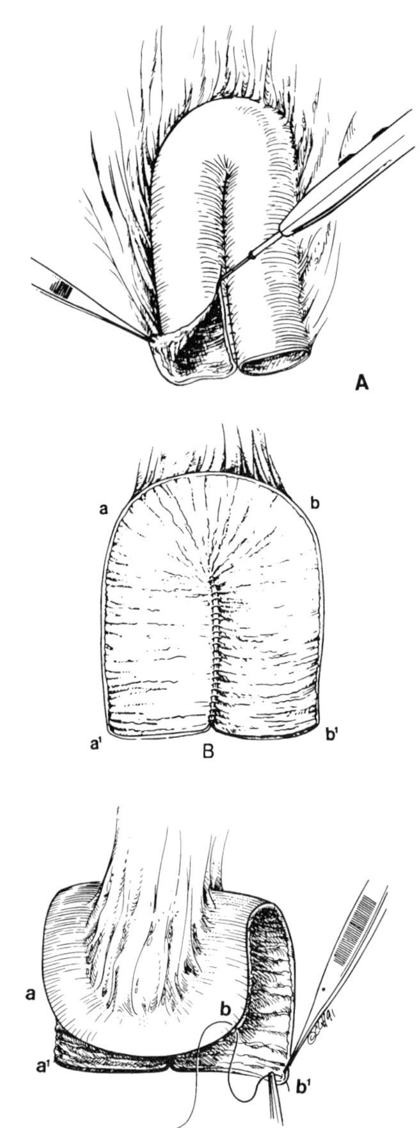

Figure 5.2 *Doubly detubularized ileum using the Kock pouch method, which provides a large, low-pressure, augmented bladder. (A) An ileal segment is folded into an inverted U, sutured along antimesenteric borders, and opened close to the suture line. (B) A second layer of suture is used to close the mucosal edges. The ileum is opened, revealing the plica. (C) Point a is sutured to a^1 and b to b^1, forming a spherical cap. All suture lines are double-layered and watertight. Reproduced with permission from Mitchell, M. and Burns, M.W. (1992)* Urinary Undiversion and Augmentation Cystoplasty. *Philadelphia, W.B. Saunders, Co.*

sigmoid colon. Ileum may be fashioned into a patch by opening along the antimesenteric border and used as a clam shell augmentation (Fig. 5.1). A more thorough detubularization involves reconfiguring the ileum, much as proposed by Willard Goodwin,[18] or using a Mainz modification[19] if a significant segment of ileum is needed (Fig. 5.2). The sigmoid colon may be treated in a similar fashion, but generally less total length is necessary due to the greater diameter. The length of bowel resected dictates the end volume of the augmentation bladder. Usually 25–30 cm of small bowel or 20–25 cm of large bowel is the minimal length required for adequate augmentation. Patient age and size influence these factors. Two simple concepts to remember include: (a) an augmentation can never be too large, but it can be too small; and (b) augmentation is performed with anticipation of the need for CIC.

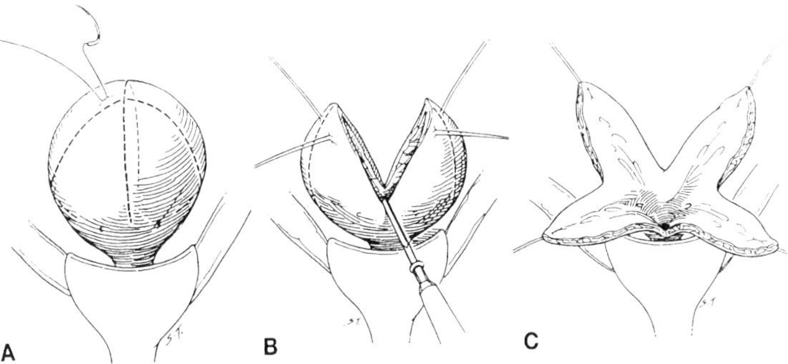

Figure 5.3 *(A) Tacking sutures are placed in each quadrant of bladder dome to facilitate handling and define proposed cystotomies. (B) Cautery is used to open bladder in sagittal and coronal plans. (C) Star configuration is completed by extending incisions to just above trigone and bladder neck. Reproduced with permission from Keating, M.A., Ludlow, J.K. and Rich, M.A. (1996)* Enterocystoplasty: the star modification. *Baltimore, Williams & Wilkins.*

A wide cystotomy is necessary to abolish detrusor pressure and prevent an hour-glass configuration to the augmentation. The bladder is incised in the midline about 1 cm from the anterior bladder neck cephalad almost until the trigone. Perpendicular incisions can be made to further increase the cystotomy and facilitate closure[20] (Fig. 5.3). An isolated segment of ileum or colon is reconfigured into a cap using two layers of absorbable suture, polyglycolic acid. The bowel segment is then anastomosed to the bladder beginning at the posterior aspect of the bladder and continuing toward the midpoint of the cystotomy, using an inner layer of running, locking suture followed by an outer layer of 3–0 polyglycolic. The suprapubic tube is brought through the wall of the bladder, anchoring with a chromic pursestring suture. The closure is continued from the midpoint of the cystotomy toward the bladder neck, again using both an inner and outer layer of absorbable suture. Occasionally, bowel needs to be sutured to itself laterally if the bladder was very small to begin with.

Colocystoplasties and continent reservoirs have been fashioned with absorbable staples.[21] The right colon and 10 cm of terminal ileum are fashioned into a pouch using the GIA stapler. The absorbable stapler is fitted into a lateral opening made in the cecum as well as into the open end of the colon, which has been folded back on itself to oppose the cecum. The stapler is fired along the antimesenteric line in order to join these two ends. The bowel is then inverted to allow for further stapling into the lumen, until the apex is traversed and the pouch completed. The posterior wall of the pouch is opened to allow for anastomosis to the bladder. This anastomosis is performed using a two-layer closure of absorbable suture. The colonic segments appear to be better suited to construction with absorbable staples than ileal segments due to their relatively larger lumen and because opposing staple lines are not required to create a pouch of adequate capacity.

The ileocecal segment can be used for augmentation, with the advantage of having the ileocecal valve to help prevent reflux, primarily when the ureters are dilated; however, resection may result in transient and, rarely, chronic diarrhea. Detubularization is critical for augmentations with cecum, ileum, and sigmoid. There are several surgical principles that warrant emphasis: (a) make the segment long enough; (b) reconfigure (detubularize) to prevent persistent contractions and to maximize volume for length of bowel resected; (c) create a tension-free anastomosis; (d) close all mesenteric windows to prevent internal herniation of intestine; (e) return the bowel to its normal anatomic position; (f) use an antireflux technique for implanting ureters; and (g) provide a continent, accessible channel for emptying.[13]

Following enterocystoplasty, adequate drainage with regular irrigation will prevent a build up of blood clot and mucus. The augmented bladder is kept on suprapubic drainage for approximately 2 to

3 weeks after surgery before a catheterization program is initiated. The suprapubic catheter is clamped and catheterization is initiated via the urethra or Mitrofanoff. Postvoid residuals can be checked by unclamping the suprapubic tube. Daily irrigation of the bladder has been shown to lessen the chance of stone formation.[22]

Techniques for preventing reflux include tunnel methods or intussuscepted intestinal nipples. Tunnels are more dependable.[23,24] The principles of adequate anchoring of the distal ureter, good backing and sufficient tunnel length-to-width ratio are essential. Reimplantation into the detrusor is preferable, but tunneling into the tinea of the cecum or sigmoid colon works as well. Tunneling into small bowel is feasible, but not as reliable.[25]

Tapering of the dilated ureter can be accomplished by several methods. Hendren has favored tailoring of the ureter,[26] whereas imbrication[27] or folding[28] can be performed if minimal narrowing is required. Psoas hitch can be necessary if the ureter is short, combining this technique with transureteroureterostomy (short ureter to long ureter) which ensures that a single, long reimplant is obtained. One good reimplant may be preferable to two marginal reimplants. The detrusor is preferable for reimplanting tapered ureters rather than large or small bowel.

Creation of a continent, catheterizable stoma is necessary if a dependable urethra for catheterization is not present. The patient with a history of posterior urethral obstruction can have residual bladder neck hypertrophy and persistent posterior urethral dilation. Exstrophy patients may have irregularities in the urethra along with sensation that precludes urethral catheterization. Some children refuse to catheterize per urethra and others find it difficult due to body habitus, manual dexterity or paraplegia.

Mitrofanoff popularized the concept of a continent, catheterizable channel employing an antirefluxing tunnel technique to achieve continence. The use of appendix, ureter,[29] tapering ileum,[30] fallopian tube,[31] or gastric tube[29] has all been described. The appendix is favored due to its consistent blood supply and anatomic location which facilitates creation of an umbilical stoma and implantation into the anterior wall of the bladder. Additional appendiceal length can be obtained by incorporating a portion of the cecum, as a tube, using a GIA stapler.[32] Spatulation of the appendix combined with of a V-flap of periumbilical skin will prevent stomal stenosis at the umbilical end. Tunneling of the appendix in the detrusor or colon is easily accomplished, and fixation of the bladder to the anterior abdominal wall ensures a straight channel. The catheterizable channel must be easy to catheterize and continent in the operating room, because difficulties encountered at this time will certainly lead to future problems.

SUMMARY

In summary, bladder augmentation using ileum or colon has been very successful for improving bladder capacity and compliance. The technical aspects have been well refined, allowing consistent results to be achieved. However, it will be extremely important to follow these patients carefully to understand the sequelae of adding intestinal mucosa to urothelial mucosa. A database summarizing all the important perimeters could be used to follow patients and facilitate long-term trends that may not be immediately apparent. Pertinent studies for patients who have undergone augmentation procedures should include metabolic studies, biochemical studies, x-ray studies, bladder function, history of infections and cystoscopic findings. The urodynamic evaluation should include assessment of bladder capacity, compliance, and leak point pressure. Past experience has shown that many years may ensue before biological changes become manifest.

REFERENCES

1. Gilchrist, R.K., Merricks, J.W., Hamlin H.H. *et al.* (1950) Construction of a substitute bladder and urethra. *Surgery, Gynecology and Obstetrics*, **90**, 752–60.
2. Bricker, E.M. (1950) Bladder substitution after pelvic evisceration. *Surgical Clinics of North America*, **30**, 1511–21.
3. Lapides, J., Diokno A.C., Gould F.R., *et al.* (1972)

Clean intermittent self-catheterization in the treatment of urinary tract disease. *Journal of Urology,* **107,** 458–61.

4. Mitchell, M.E., Kolb, T.B. and Backes, D.J. (1986) Intestinocystoplasty in combination with clean intermittent catheterization in the management of vesical dysfunction. *Journal of Urology,* **136,** 288–91.
5. Mitchell, M.E. and Piser, J.A. (1987) Intestinocystoplasty and total bladder replacement in children and young adults: follow up in 129 cases. *Journal of Urology,* **138,** 579–84.
6. King, L.R., Webster G.D. and Bertram, R.A. (1987) Experience with bladder reconstruction in children. *Journal of Urology,* **138**, 1002–6.
7. Hendren, W.H. and Hendren, R.B. (1990) Bladder augmentation experience with 129 children and young adults. *Journal of Urology,* **144**, 445–53.
8. Kuss, R., Bitker, M., Camey, M. *et al.* (1970) Indications and early and late results of intestinocystoplasty: a review of 185 cases. *Journal of Urology,* **103**, 53–63.
9. Smith, R.B., VanCangh, P., Skinner, D.G. *et al.* (1977) Augmentation enterocystoplasty: a critical review. *Journal of Urology,* **118**, 35–9.
10. Malone, P.S., Ransley, P.G. and Kiely, E.M. (1990) Preliminary report: the antegrade continence enema. *Lancet*, **336**, 1217–18.
11. Koyle, M.A., Kaji, D.M., Duque M. *et al.* (1995) The Malone antegrade continence enema for neurogenic and structural fecal incontinence and constipation. *Journal of Urology,* **154**, 759–61.
12. Mitrofanoff, P. (1980) Cystostomic continente transappendiculaire dans le treatment des vessies neurogiques. *Chirurgie Pediatrique,* **21**, 297–305.
13. Mitchell, M.E. and Burns, M.W. (1992) Urinary undiversion and augmentation cystoplasty. In *Clinical Pediatric Urology,* 3rd edn, Kelalis, P., King, L. and Belman, B. (eds.), W.B. Saunders, Philadelphia, 904–19.
14. McGuire, E.J., Woodside, J.R. and Borden, T.A. (1983) Upper urinary tract deterioration in patients with myelodysplasia and detrusor hypertonia: a follow-up study. *Journal of Urology,* **129**, 823–6.
15. Horowitz, M., Kuhr, C.S. and Mitchell, M.E. (1995) The Mitrofanoff catheterizable channel: patient acceptance. *Journal of Urology,* **153,** 771–2.
16. Scheidler, D.M., Brito, C.G., Rink, R.C. *et al.* (1989) Insight into bladder rupture following lower urinary tract reconstruction. *Journal of Urology,* **141**, 102A.
17. Bauer, S.B., Hendren, W.H., Kozakewich, H. *et al.* (1992) Perforation of the augmented bladder. *Journal of Urology,* **148,** 699–703.
18. Goodwin, W.E., Turner, R.D. and Winter, C.C. (1958) Results of ileocystoplasty. *Journal of Urology,* **80**, 461–6.
19. Thuroff, J.W., Alken, P., Riedmiller, H. *et al.* (1988) A hundred cases of Mainz pouch: continuing experience and evaluation. *Journal of Urology,* **130**, 283–8.
20. Keating, M.A., Ludlow, J.K. and Rich, M.A. (1996) Enterocystoplasty: the star modification. *Journal of Urology,* **155**, 1723–5.
21. Kirsch, A.J., Olsson, C.A. and Hensle, T.W. (1996) Pediatric continent reservoirs and colocystoplasties created with absorbable staples. *Journal of Urology,* **156**, 614–17.
22. Nurse, D.E., McInerney, P.D., Thomas, P.J. *et al.* (1996) Stones in enterocystoplasties. *British Journal of Urology,* **77**, 684–7.
23. LeDuc, A. and Camey, M. (1979) A procedure for avoiding reflux in uretero-ileal implantations during enterocystoplasty. *Journal of Urology/Nephrology,* (Paris) **85**, 449–54.
24. Gregoir, W. (1969) Surgical management of congenital reflux and primary megaureter. *International Urology,* **24**, 502–26.
25. Lilien, O.M. and Camey, M. (1984) Twenty-five year experience with replacement of the human bladder (Camey procedure). *Journal of Urology,* **132,** 886–91.
26. Hendren, W.H. (1969) Operative repair of megaureter in children. *Journal of Urology,* **101**, 491–507.
27. Starr, A. (1979) Ureteral plication: a new concept in ureteral tailoring for megaureter. *Investigative Urology,* **17**, 153–8.
28. Kalicinski, Z.H., Kansy, J., Kotarbinska, B. *et al.* (1977) Surgery of megaureters – modification of Hendren's operation. *Journal of Pediatric Surgery,* **12**, 183–8.
29. Mitchell, M.E. (1991) Gastrocystoplasty and bladder replacement with stomach. In *Operative Urology*, Marshall, F. (ed.), W.B. Saunders, Philadelphia, 251–8.

30. Lobe, T.E. (1986) Conversion of an ileal conduit into a neourethral enteroplication for urinary continence: tips and proper construction. *Journal of Pediatric Surgery,* **21**, 1040–1.
31. Duckett, J.W. and Snyder H.M. (1986) Continent urinary diversion: variations on the Mitrofanoff principle. *Journal of Urology,* **136**, 58–62.
32. Burns, M.W. and Mitchell, M.E. (1990) Tips on constructing the Mitrofanoff continent appendiceal stoma. *Contemporary Urology,* **2**, 10–12.

6

Gastrocystoplasty

RICHARD W GRADY AND MICHAEL E MITCHELL

INTRODUCTION

The use of large and small bowel in the reconstruction of the lower urinary tract has resulted in a variety of long-term problems. These include difficulty with catheterization and emptying due to mucus production, chronic metabolic acidosis secondary to urine electrolyte reabsorption through bowel mucosa with its subsequent effects on growth and development, and risk for malignant degeneration[1–3] (see Chapter 7). These issues are particularly relevant to children who are candidates for urinary reconstruction which must last a lifetime and still provide metabolic homeostasis for optimal growth and development.

Largely because of these concerns, various investigators have attempted to find the best material for bladder replacement. In 1956, Sinaiko described the use of stomach for urinary diversion in a canine model.[4] Use of gastric antrum was later reported by Leong and Ong who popularized gastric bladder replacement after cystectomy.[5] In the USA use of stomach for bladder augmentation was studied in an animal model by Rudick in the 1970s and by Mitchell and coworkers at Indiana University where interest was focused on the use of stomach in the setting of chronic metabolic acidosis and azotemia.[6,7] Gastrocystoplasty in a canine model with chronic renal failure was successful in partially treating chronic metabolic acidosis. Gastric bladder augmentation in azotemic animals also promoted acid–base homeostasis when compared to controls with colocystoplasty that demonstrated increased chloride, ammonium, sodium, and phosphorus absorption from urine.[7] Several large clinical studies based on the surgical technique of the wedge and antral gastrocystoplasty have now been reported.[8–10] These series illustrate the advantages of gastric bladder augmentation as well as the complications associated with this technique (Table 6.1).

PHYSIOLOGY OF GASTRIC AUGMENTATION: A PERSISTENT PHYSIOLOGY

The native stomach functions as an organ with secretory and mechanical (storage and emptying)

Table 6.1 *Advantages and disadvantages of the use of stomach*

Advantages	Disadvantages
Net secretion of hydrogen and chloride ions	Metabolic electrolyte disorders/alkalosis
Less viscous/more soluble mucus	Hematuria–dysuria syndrome (36%)
Decreased incidence of UTI	Bladder/gastric ulceration/perforation (rare)
Decreased incidence of stone formation	Gastrointestinal complications (rare)
Favorable fibromuscular properties	Possible tumor potential (unknown)
Available tissue in most patients	
Facilitates tunnels for continence	

properties. It is responsible for the acid production necessary for the digestion of food. It is also intimately involved in the production of peptides which act locally and at distant sites in the body. These include intrinsic factor and pepsinogens. Intrinsic factor binds with vitamin B12 to assist in the absorption of this vitamin in the distal ileum. Secretion of this factor is driven by gastric acid production. Similarly, pepsinogens are released by acid stimulation as well as by vagal nerve stimulation. These are converted to proteases in an acid environment (pH <5.0) and are released by chief and mucous cells in the body, antrum, and pylorus of the stomach.

Acid production arises from the parietal cells in the form of hydrochloric acid. Parietal cells secrete acid in response to several stimuli: gastrin production in the antrum of the stomach and direct vagal stimulation via muscarinic receptors in the parietal cells. Histamine, amino acids and peptides, and gastric distension also trigger acid production from the parietal cells. Fat and hyperosmolar contents decrease acid production. Inhibitory responses are, in part, controlled in a paracrine and local endocrine fashion by factors such as glucagon, gastrointestinal peptide (GIP), and vasoactive intestinal peptide (VIP) (Fig. 6.1).

The gastric lining of the stomach is protected from this acid production by an alkaline mucous barrier which arises from the parietal cells of the stomach. Parietal cells are involved in electrolyte

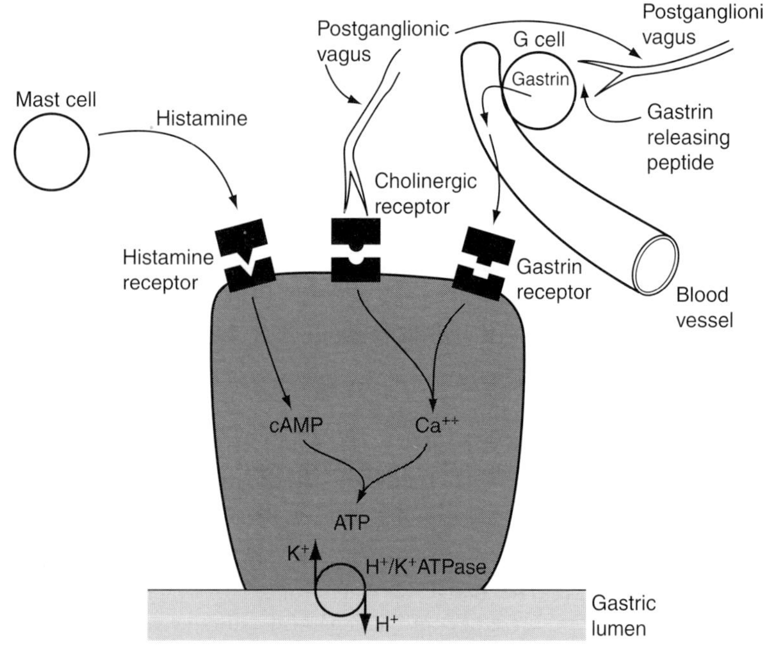

Figure 6.1 *Diagram of a parietal cell in the stomach. Acid production from this cell is caused by various mechanisms, including stimulation from histamine, acetylcholine, and gastrin. The activated receptors act through Ca^{2+} or cAMP to drive an ATP-dependent hydrogen–potassium ion pump at the gastric lumen. Reproduced with permission from Figure 30.5 in Pappas, T.N. (1997) Stomach. In* Textbook of Surgery. The Biologic Basis of Modern Surgical Practice, *15th edn. D.J. Sabiston and H.K. Lyerly (eds.), Philadelphia, W.B. Saunders, Co: 847.*

transport and actively secrete bicarbonate which is incorporated into the mucous layer. They also transport sodium, potassium, chloride, and bicarbonate into the stomach. This layer also prevents back-exchange of hydrogen and sodium ions because of its buffering capacity.

Placement of the stomach into contact with urine does not affect its ability to secrete acid. Early experimental studies in a canine model by Sinaiko and by Leong reveal a continued ability of the stomach to secrete acid in this environment.[4,5] Later studies by Piser, Mitchell, and coworkers also demonstrate a net secretion of chloride ions into the urine of bladders augmented with stomach.[7] Because the intercellular tight junctions of stomach are somewhat like those in the bladder the net transmural resorption of water is small when compared to the epithelial lining of small and large intestine.[11] The net ion flux of a gastric flap results in net hydrogen, sodium, and chloride secretion into urine. In contrast, urinary reconstruction with large or small intestine results in net reabsorption of ammonia , hydrogen, potassium, sodium, and chloride ions to produce a pattern of hyperchloremic metabolic acidosis (Fig. 6.2).[12] This metabolic consequence of using large and small bowel is well recognized. In the majority of patients the metabolic effects of enteric augmentation are manifest by a decrease in total body buffering capacity. However, in children and patients with altered renal or hepatic reserve, more significant clinical evidence of these metabolic effects can be seen usually as decreased somatic growth, clinical acidosis, and hyperammonemia respectively. Patients augmented with stomach less often exhibit any clinical evidence of the metabolic effects associated with stomach, although a hypochloremic, hyponatremic metabolic alkalosis is possible, particularly in the patient with salt and acid loss (i.e., vomiting, salt-wasting nephropathy).[13]

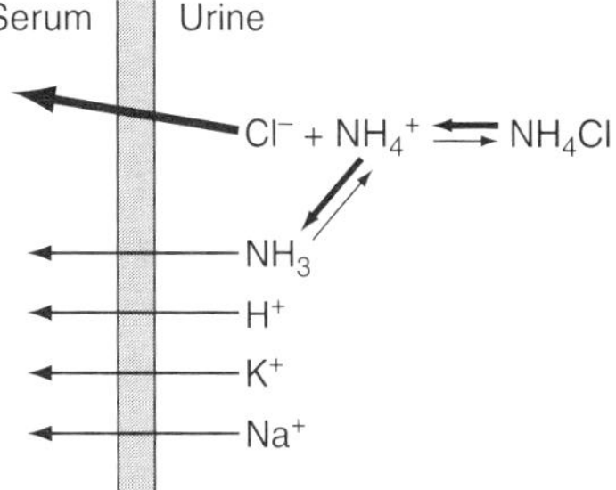

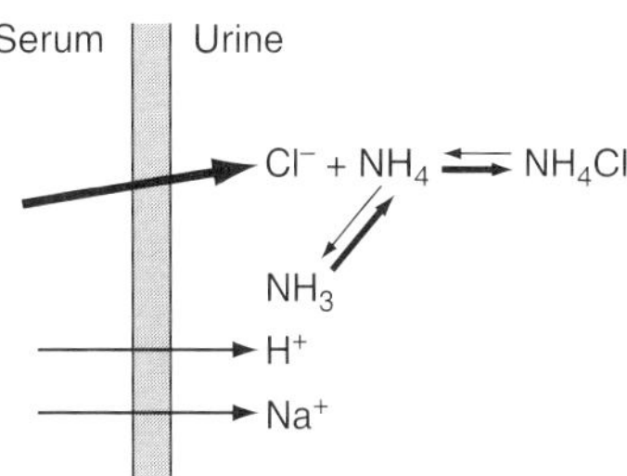

Figure 6.2 *Ion flux. Diagram depicting ion shifts through the luminal activity of (a) small and large intestines and (b) stomach when these segments are used for bladder augmentation. Large and small intestinal segments cause a net ion shift of hydrogen (H^+), potassium (K^+), and sodium (Na^+) ions, and ammonia (NH_3) from urine to serum. In contrast, ion shifts associated with gastric segments result in active secretion of chloride (Cl^-) and hydrogen ions into urine. Reproduced with permission from Figure 17.1 in Mitchell, M.A. and Horowitz, M. (1995) The gastric continent urinary reseroir. In* Urinary Diversion, Scientific Foundation and Clinical Practice. *G.D. Webster and B. Goldwasser (eds.). Oxford, Isis Medical Media.*

To determine the persistence of gastric physiology of augmented segments taken from the body of the stomach, Bogaert and coworkers performed a prospective study of children who had undergone a gastrocystoplasty between 6 months and 4.5 years prior to the study. The median postoperative period was 2 years. In a fasting state, urinary pH was neutral in these patients and serum gastrin levels were within normal limits. However, after ingestion of food, urinary pH decreased and serum gastrin levels rose. Pharmacologic manipulation with histamine-2 antagonists and anticholinergic agents decreased acid secretion by the augmentation but did not affect serum gastrin levels. Interestingly, gastric bladder distension did not increase acid production by the augmented segment and did not affect serum gastrin levels in these patients. Bogaert *et al.* concluded that the cyclic acid production relating to diet may be partially inhibited by acid ingestion with meals to decrease gastrin production in the gastric antrum.

Overall, however, the gastric body was found to retain its native properties and continue to act like stomach, even in a urinary environment.[14]

ADVANTAGES OF USING STOMACH

Electrolyte balance

Stomach offers the unique advantage of net secretion of hydrogen and chloride ions when compared to other gastrointestinal segments.[15] Acid-loading studies performed in a canine gastrocystoplasty model reveal a remarkable resistance to the development of systemic acidosis in these animals.[7] In these acid-loading experiments, the animals also demonstrate less weight loss than either control subjects or dogs that have undergone colocystoplasty.[16] The same metabolic patterns are seen in human subjects. In clinical series, patients are noted to have a slight decrease in serum chloride levels and increase in serum bicarbonate levels following antral or corporal gastric augmentation regardless of underlying renal function.[17,18] In a series of 23 patients reported by Sheldon *et al.*, no patient developed acidosis, alkalosis, or alterations in serum chloride levels. Further, acid secretion from the gastric augmentation was sufficient in five patients with chronic renal failure to obviate their need for bicarbonate supplementation.[19]

Ammonia metabolism is also significantly affected with gastrointestinal augmentation of the urinary tract. Chloride reabsorption by large and small intestinal segments exposed to urine increases hydrogen ion reabsorption in the form of ammonium (NH_4^+) because ammonia chloride acts as one of the primary buffers in urine (Fig. 6.2).[20] To add to this, ammonium ions may also drive chloride ion (Cl^-) reabsorption.[21] These increased serum ammonia levels are easily compensated in healthy patients. However, patients with altered hepatic function can be overwhelmed with an increased ammonia burden and develop portasystemic encephalopathy. Gastric bladder augmentation provides a means to avoid this complication in patients with liver dysfunction because of the favorable electrolyte resorptive pattern of stomach (Fig. 6.2).[13]

Mucus production

All segments of the gastrointestinal tract will continue to produce mucus after incorporation into the lower urinary tract. Stomach offers the advantage of less viscous and more soluble mucus production. This quality allows catheter drainage with smaller-lumen catheters. Mucus from colonic and ileal augmentation is notably thicker and more flocculent and often requires active irrigation to achieve adequate drainage of urine. Consequently, mucus from these segments has been implicated in bladder outlet obstruction, as a nidus for bladder calculus formation, and in catheter occlusion resulting in renal impairment in at least one patient.[22] Catheter obstruction from mucus can also cause bladder rupture by creating chronic urinary retention and subsequent bladder overdistension. In contrast, patients augmented with stomach will often demonstrate grossly clear urine with no visible mucus sediment even on spun urine samples.[13] Mucus production from gastric segments has been reported by some investigators to be less than other segments,[22,23] whereas others have noted no difference in quantity.[12]

Urinary tract infections

Patients undergoing bladder augmentation with gastrointestinal segments are prone to urinary tract infection. Asymptomatic bacteriuria is nearly universal in this patient population, due in part to the prevalence of clean intermittent catheterization. Decreased mucus production and acid production by the gastric augmentation offer theoretical advantages which should lower the incidence of urinary tract infection. Experiments in a uremic dog model have shown that gastric augmentation is superior to colonic augmentation in preventing or reducing the incidence of urinary tract infection.[16,24] Long-term studies in a rat model have also shown a decreased incidence of urinary tract infection.[25,26] In a large clinical study of 231 patients, Hollensbe and coworkers at Indiana University noted a decreased incidence of both symptomatic cystitis and febrile urinary tract infections in patients augmented with stomach. In this series of patients who had undergone bladder augmentation, symptomatic cystitis was documented in 22.7% of the patients after ileocystoplasty versus 8% after gastrocystoplasty. Febrile infection rates were 13.6% and 10.8% respectively. So, while the difference in the incidence of febrile infections is not statistically significant, the rate of cystitis is clearly decreased by the use of stomach in a human population.[27]

Stone formation

Bladder calculus formation has been recognized as a common complication of enterocystoplasty, with some series reporting rates as high as 52%.[28,29] The vast majority of these stones are composed of struvite, although apatite and ammonium urate stones have been reported. All segments of small or large bowel are noted to predispose to the formation of bladder calculi. However, stomach is a notable exception. Theoretically, stones which form in an acidic environment could form in a gastric urinary reservoir or augmented bladder. However, stone formation has been reported after gastrocystoplasty in only one patient to date, with the report of a uric acid stone in a 3-year-old girl with cloacal exstrophy 7 months after gastrocystoplasty.[30] Factors implicated in the decreased incidence of stone formation associated with gastric bladder augmentation include decreased mucus production, decreased episodes of cystitis, and urinary acid secretion.[31] In fact, Goodwin proposed replacement of the renal pelvis with stomach in a patient with severe recurrent stone disease years ago.[32]

Fibromuscular properties

Stomach musculature is similar to that of native bladder. It is composed of three layers – an outer longitudinal layer, a middle circular layer, and an inner oblique layer – which fuse as one layer.[31] This anatomic arrangement is felt to permit improved emptying of the augmented bladder without catheterization. Ganeson, Mitchell, and coworkers reported a series of 18 patients who achieved urinary continence and the ability to empty their bladders without catheterization after gastrocystoplasty and artificial urinary sphincter placement.[33] Urodynamic studies by various investigators have also found the gastric segment to demonstrate excellent compliance and capacity.[34–6] In a series reported from Boston Children's Hospital, overall bladder capacity increased 220% (range of 20% to 750%) and maximum intravesical pressures during filling decreased an average of 32%, with a mean pressure of 32 cmH20.[34] Of note, rhythmic, uninhibited contractions occur on filling the bladder in some patients after gastrocystoplasty. This finding is attributed to the underlying peristaltic activity of stomach which generates small coordinated contractions as compared to the mass tubular contraction seen in other bowel segments. These contractions are usually first observed with the bladder partially full and increase in amplitude as capacity is approached. They may necessitate re-augmentation if the pressures place the upper urinary tracts at risk for deterioration of function.[37] However, compared to the use of other enteric segments where detubularization of the augmented segment is of critical importance in achieving appropriate urodynamic properties, the stomach does not contract in a tubular fashion and lends itself to spherical construction. The gastric pedicle also facilitates spherical bladder reconstruction, which results in efficient storage of fluid under low wall tension.[38] In many patients, stomach also demonstrates a capacity to distend (increase surface area) with time, a phenomenon which does not occur with all patients with other forms of enterocystoplasty.[34,35]

The intrinsic structure of the gastric wall also lends itself to submucosal tunneling techniques because the submucosa and muscularis readily separate to form a submucosal plane.[39] The importance of this characteristic cannot be overemphasized in reconstructive cases in which a continent stoma and/or antireflux mechanism must be created. To prevent stenosis at the gastric mucosal interface of the tunnel, it is helpful to create a nipple mechanism at the end of the tunnel. This prevents a circumferential anastomosis.

Renal function/hydronephrosis

Most studies report stable or improved renal function after gastrocystoplasty along with improvement or stabilization of hydronephrosis.[40–42] In a study of

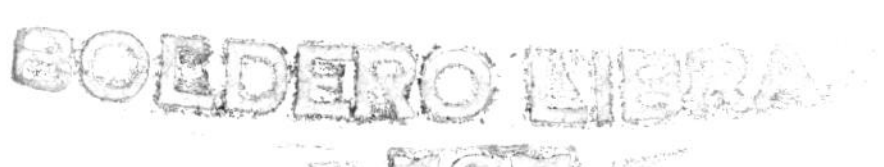

28 children with either normal (n=10) or impaired (n=18) renal function, Kogan and coworkers found stable renal function in all patients at a median follow-up of 2 years. Further, hydronephrosis either decreased or disappeared entirely in all the patients with this preoperative finding (n=18). These investigators also noted a marked improvement in the subjective impression of well-being in the children who underwent gastrocystoplasty.[41]

SURGICAL TECHNIQUES USING STOMACH

Metabolic alkalosis

Clinically significant metabolic alkalosis has been reported in approximately 6–25% of patients who have undergone gastric bladder reconstruction.[31,42] This metabolic derangement is a direct result of the secretory nature of gastric epithelium. It occurs largely because of excessive secretion of hydrogen chloride and potassium into urine and results in a hyponatremic, hypokalemic, hypochloremic metabolic alkalosis. This pattern is similar to that seen in upper intestinal obstruction such as pyloric stenosis or duodenal webs. Systemic alkalosis can present with nonspecific symptoms involving the neuromuscular, cardiovascular, and pulmonary systems. These symptoms can include malaise, fatigue, lethargy, decreased responsiveness, and/or cardiac dysrhythmias.[43] Patients with a tendency to waste salts and fluids are most at risk for this complication. These include patients with salt-wasting nephropathy or short bowel syndrome.[12] In otherwise normal patients, acute episodes of gastroenteritis can also result in severe metabolic alkalosis.[18] Consequently, this complication has been reported in patients with both normal and impaired renal function.[42,44]

Other factors involved in the development of this phenomenon include hypergastrinemia. This has been reported in some patients and causes increased gastric acid output into the augmented bladder.[42] Detection of elevated serum gastrin levels in these patients can potentially be treated by weak oral acid ingestion such as ascorbic acid or cola beverages.[45] The source of gastrin secretion has not yet been elucidated but is presumed to arise from the stomach and act in an endocrine fashion on the gastric augment. However, chronic retention of the gastric bladder may also result in increased serum gastrin levels.[46] Severe potassium depletion can also sustain and worsen metabolic alkalosis by increasing the rate of renal tubular bicarbonate reabsorption. Furthermore, decreased serum sodium levels may cause increased aldosterone production with resultant renal potassium loss.[47] Glassberg reported on two patients who required high-dose oral potassium chloride supplementation to correct a refractory metabolic alkalosis associated with hypokalemia, and Nakagawa described a case of severe metabolic alkalosis following gastrocystoplasty with an associated serum potassium of 1.6 mEq/L which was successfully treated with intravenous and oral potassium chloride supplementation.[43,47] Severe dehydration can also be an inciting or aggravating factor by causing increased aldosterone production, which leads to increased potassium excretion and hypokalemia.[47] These patients will require saline administration to correct the metabolic abnormality in conjunction with other measures.[43]

Hematuria/dysuria syndrome

Hematuria and dysuria syndrome (HDS) may arise from the acid secretory activity of the gastric segment causing breakdown of the normal glycosaminoglycan (GAG) layer of the bladder. Urethral pain, skin irritation, hematuria, and dysuria comprise the major symptoms of this syndrome.[48] This well-known complication of gastric augmentation severely affects approximately 5% of patients who undergo this procedure. However, some investigators note the transient occurrence of this syndrome in almost all patients who undergo gastric augmentation. Fortunately, in the vast majority HDS is mild, temporary, and easily treated.[31] In the series from Children's Hospital in Seattle, 36% of patients reported this syndrome; approximately 50% of these required medication. Eighty-two per cent of patients with gastrocystoplasty required no therapy. However, removal of the gastric segment may be required if medical management fails to control the symptoms. Patients at higher risk of developing HDS include those with urinary incontinence, sensate urethras, and possibly those with renal insufficiency and inadequate urine salt concentration to buffer acid production by the gastric segment.[48] However, the syndrome has been reported in continent patients with normal renal function as well.[31] HDS has also been reported with the use of gastric antrum to augment the bladder but appears to occur less often with this segment compared to the body of the stomach.[36] Treatment usually consists of H2 blockade. Only 8% of the patients in one series required chronic medical management.[47] In this patient group, serum gastrin levels should also be assessed. If the gastrin level is elevated, initiation of mild oral acid therapy (i.e., cola beverages with meals) may also help control the symptoms.[45] Instalation of baking soda into the bladder may also relieve symptoms.[31] Omeprazole is not recommended in the chronic treatment of this syndrome if gastrin levels are elevated, because it will also elevate serum gastrin levels.[49] Theoretically, this medication should also not be used for extended periods because of concerns of tumor formation.[50] It is interesting to note that cystoscopic examination in the patients with HDS has not revealed any evidence of ulceration in either native bladder or gastric segment.[36]

Bladder ulceration and perforation

Bladder ulceration has been reported in animal models and in humans following gastrocystoplasty.[51–3] Gastric augmentation appears prone to ulceration and/or perforation with urinary diversion or oliguric states. Reinberg described perforation of the gastric segment of a defunctionalized bladder after gastric augmentation and felt that this occurred secondary to the lack of buffering by urine.[54] Animal studies reveal that dogs more readily develop perforations if the gastrocystoplasty is diverted of urine. Indeed, oliguria or anuria produces a rapid effect on both gastric and bladder epithelium in this model in the form of peptic and bladder ulceration.[51,52] Evidence of cystitis in the native bladder segment is also more prominent when urine is diverted or poorly buffered, as in the case of polyuric patients with poor tubular concentrating capacity. Therefore, urine has a protective effect on the epithelium which probably results from the inherent buffering capacity of urine (dependent on urinary salt concentration) but may also be a result of other factors such as the ability of urine to decrease antral gastrin production.[55] Patients should be placed on H2 blockers or proton pump antagonists if they are oliguric or undergo temporary urinary diversion after gastrocystoplasty.[56] Delayed perforation after gastrocystoplasty, however, has been rare and occurs much less commonly than with most other gastrointestinal segments.[31]

Gastrointestinal complications

Transient early satiety is commonly seen in the first few weeks following gastrocystoplasty. However, more severe complications have been reported much less frequently. Potential complications following gastric resection include delayed gastric emptying, feeding intolerance, food aversion with subsequent weight loss, dumping syndrome, and esophagitis. In one series from the Hospital for Sick Children in Toronto, five patients developed failure to thrive approximately 4 to 6 months following gastrocystoplasty. All five patients were managed with nutritional and pharmacologic intervention depending on the underlying problem. This has been an extremely rare occurrence in our experience and may reflect a technical problem with either excessive gastric resection or partial obstruction of the duodenum by inadequate mobilization of the right gastroepiploic artery. The authors state that patients with chronic renal failure may be at higher risk for developing gastrointestinal complications because these patients are already prone to nausea, vomiting, anorexia, and poor weight gain.[57] These symptoms are known to be aggravated by gastric surgery in azotemic patients.[58]

Tumour formation

Long-term studies of gastrointestinal augmentation or reconstruction of the urinary tract have demonstrated malignant degeneration of augmented tissue in patients who have undergone augmentation with ileum or large intestine.[59] Animal studies in a rat model suggest that gastric segments may also have potential for malignant degeneration. Investigators found bladder papillomas at the junctional zone between bladder and stomach in five of 15 rats 18 months after gastric augmentation.[60] Follow-up studies in this same model (Long–Evans female rat) also revealed hyperplastic or metaplastic changes in the gastrointestinal patches or urothelium of all the animals that had been augmented. Although some demonstrated cellular pleomorphism characteristic of malignancy, no tumor displayed invasive properties or other evidence of true malignancy.[25] These findings have been corroborated by other investigators.[61,62] Despite these findings, no evidence of malignant degeneration of a gastric segment exists to date. The longest follow-up of patients who have undergone gastric augmentation is from patients who have undergone antral gastrocystoplasty, with a mean follow-up of 16 years. Biopsies of these patients reveal mild to moderate degrees of inflammation, with atrophy in four of 18 patients.[36] Because of this unrealized concern of malignant degeneration, most authors recommend a protocol of chronic surveillance cystoscopy and biopsies starting 7 to 10 years after augmentation.[31]

Further discussion of complications resulting from incorporation of stomach in the urinary tract is presented in Chapter 7.

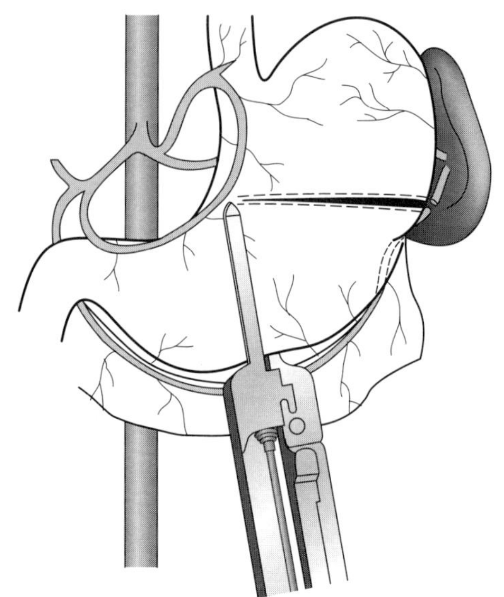

Figure 6.3 *Dividing the omentum. To harvest the gastric segment, the greater omentum must be divided, with care taken to preserve the gastroiepiploic vessels. This can be done with electrocautery as depicted in this diagram. Reproduced with permission from Figure 2 in Sumfest, J.M. and Mitchell, M.E. (1994) Gastrocystoplasty in children.* European Urology, ***25***, *89, Karger, Basel.*

TECHNIQUE OF WEDGE GASTROCYSTOPLASTY

Preoperative patient preparation consists of a clear liquid diet for approximately 24–48 hours before surgery. Magnesium citrate is given the day before surgery. More rigorous bowel evacuation regimens are reserved for patients with severe constipation. Intravenous antibiotics are started the night prior to surgery if the patient has bacterial colonization of the urinary tract. Otherwise, antibiotic therapy is initiated at the time of surgery. H2 receptor antagonists are also started at this time and continued for at least 1 month after surgery.

A longitudinal incision is made from the symphysis pubis to the xiphoid process. A wedge-shaped segment of stomach is then harvested from the midportion of the greater curvature of the stomach. This segment will contain mostly corpus. The size of the segment to be used will depend on the size of the patient and on the anticipated procedure – augmentation versus continent reservoir. The length of stomach taken, as measured along the greater curvature, is usually between 8 and 14cm. The greater omentum is incised several centimeters away from the greater curvature to preserve the omentum and to avoid compromising the blood supply to the gastric segment (Fig. 6.3). Omental vessels should be suture ligated. Stapling devices can be used to isolate this segment to reduce the potential for peritoneal spill of gastric contents (Fig. 6.4). The segment removed should not extend all the way across the stomach but should instead avoid the lesser curvature to prevent injury to the branches of the vagus nerve. When basing the flap on the right gastroepiploic artery, branches of the left gastric artery near the lesser curvature need to be ligated near the apex of the gastric segment before preparing the pedicle to reduce traction on the short gastric and splenic vessels (Fig. 6.5). Because the watershed area between the right and left gastroepiploic vessels

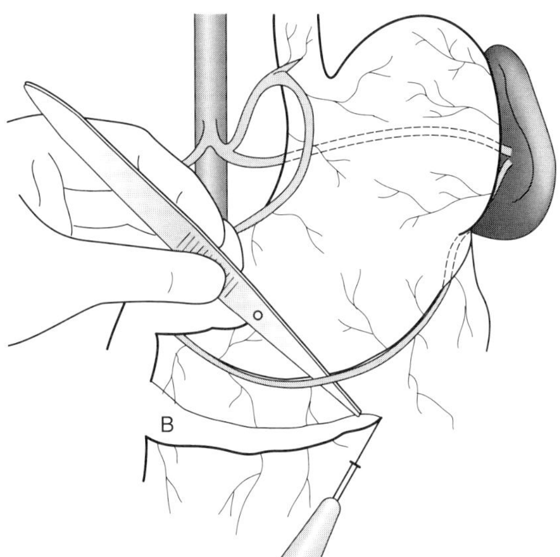

Figure 6.4 *Stapling across the stomach. The use of gastrointestinal stapling devices simplifies the isolation of the gastric segment. A wedge-shaped segment taken from the body of the stomach avoids problems associated with using the antral segment of the stomach. Reproduced with permission from Figure 3 in Sumfest, J.M. and Mitchell, M.E. (1994) Gastrocystoplasty in children.* European Urology, ***25****, 89, Karger, Basel.*

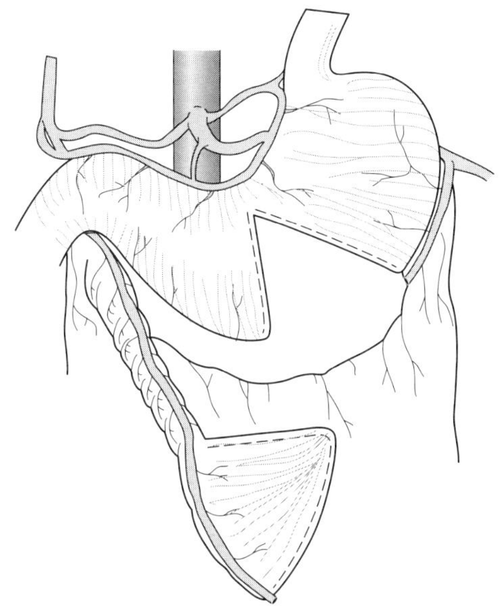

Figure 6.5 *Avoid the lesser curvature during isolation and dissection of the gastric segment. During isolation of the gastric segment, care is taken not to include the lesser curvature of the stomach, which would cause damage to the vagal nerve resulting in gastric emptying problems. Reproduced with permission from Bagli, D. and Mitchell, M.E. (1995) Current applications of gastric segments in reconstructive urology. (eds: Nieh, P., Libertino, J.A.)* Atlas of the Urologic Clinics of North America, ***3****(2), 1.*

usually occurs to the left of the midline, the gastric pedicle is most often based on the right gastroepiploic artery. The right gastroepiploic artery also offers a more constant blood supply in the majority of patients. Patients with cloacal exstrophy are a notable exception to this finding. Papaverine may be applied to the pedicle while it is being harvested to prevent vasospasm. Bissada and Bissada recommend temporary atraumatic occlusion of the gastroepiploic vessel to assess the adequacy of circulation prior to dividing the gastroepiploic vessels.[63] We have not found this maneuver to be necessary.

An oblique wedge resection may be used in those patients who have a long greater stomach curvature which produces a 'droop.' This maneuver avoids the need for a gastric closure but also tends to foreshorten the vascular pedicle.[12] If a 'classic' wedge resection is performed, the staples are removed from the stomach along its anterior layer. The stomach anastomosis is then performed in two layers.

The gastric wedge is brought down into the pelvis by creating a window through the mesocolon and omentum of the small bowel (Fig. 6.6). The pedicle should be anchored in the retroperitoneum to prevent torsion of the vessels. After the wedge has been brought into the pelvis, it should be isolated with towels and then opened and irrigated with saline and antibiotic solution. Meticulous removal of all staples is required at this time to avoid niduses of stone formation in the augmented bladder. Ureteral reimplantation, if necessary, is usually performed at this time with the bladder open. The ureters may be reimplanted into the native bladder or gastric segment (Fig. 6.7). A ureteral nipple technique should be used if the ureter is reimplanted into the gastric segment to reduce the incidence of ureteral stenosis (Figs. 6.8 and 6.9). The gastric segment is then widely anastomosed

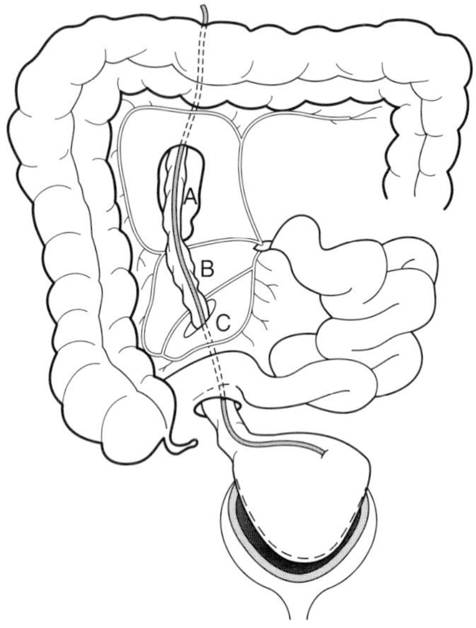

Figure 6.6 *Bringing the gastric wedge into the pelvis. The gastric segment can be brought down to the pelvis retroperitoneally by creating openings in the transverse mesocolon, root of the small bowel mesentery, and ileocecal mesentery, as depicted in this diagram. This decreases the risk for intestinal wrapping or strangulation around the gastroepiploic pedicle. Reproduced with permission from Figure 4 in Sumfest, J.M. and Mitchell, M.E. (1994) Gastrocystoplasty in children.* European Urology, ***25***, *89.*

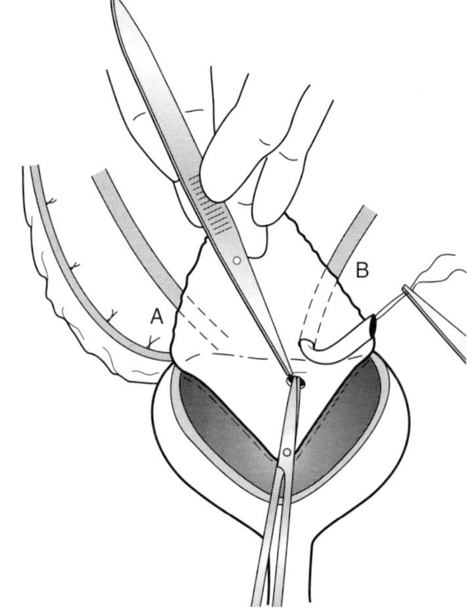

Figure 6.7 *Ureteral reimplantation into gastric segment. Submucosal tunnels can be developed in the gastric segment in a fashion analogous to submucosal tunnel development in the native bladder. This allows the ureters to be brought into either the native bladder or the gastric segment during gastrocystoplasty. Reproduced with permission from Figure 6 in Sumfest, J.M. and Mitchell, M.E. (1994) Gastrocystoplasty in children.* European Urology, ***25***, *89.*

to the bivalved native bladder in two layers with absorbable suture material in a running fashion.

Some authors have recently advocated the use of other bowel segments in conjunction with stomach in the construction of urinary reservoirs or bladder augmentation. The theoretical and apparent clinical advantage is that of achieving salt and electrolyte homeostasis by balancing electrolyte and water reabsorption by intestine with salt excretion by the gastric segment.[64]

PATIENT SELECTION FOR GASTROCYSTOPLASTY

Because of the unique advantages of stomach, it is particularly suited to certain patient populations.

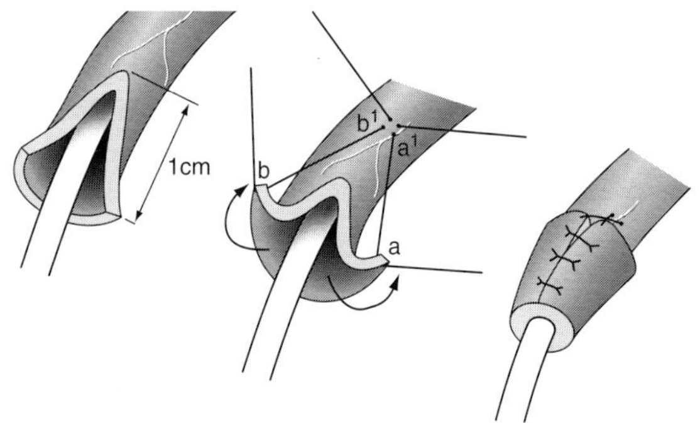

Figure 6.8 *Nipple mechanism. Ureteral spatulation technique to reduce the incidence of ureteral reflux and ureteral stenosis. Reproduced with permission from Figure 1 in Sagalowsky, A. (1996) Early results with split-cuff nipple ureteral reimplants in urinary diversion.* Journal of Urology, ***154***, *2028.*

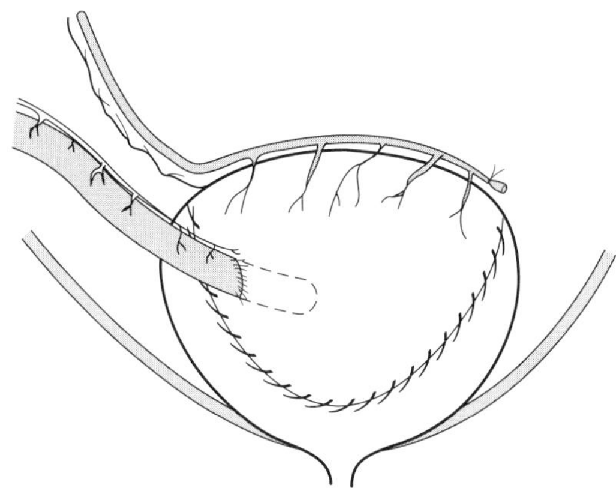

Figure 6.9 *Construction of an appendix nipple mechanism into the gastric segment to create a continent catheterizable (Mitrofanoff) channel. An appendicovesicostomy or other derivation of the Mitrofanoff principle can be applied to the gastric segment because of the facility with which submucosal dissection can be performed in the gastric segment, as depicted in this diagram. Reproduced with permission from Figure 7 in Sumfest, J.M. and Mitchell, M.E. (1994) Gastrocystoplasty in children.* European Urology, ***25***, *89.*

Routine use of the stomach to augment bladder, on the other hand, has not come to pass because of the unique disadvantages that stomach creates when placed into the urinary tract.

As previously indicated, stomach is ideally suited for use in patients with significant renal insufficiency and/or metabolic acidosis. The electrolyte transport mechanism of gastric mucosa facilitates the secretion of acid into urine to correct the metabolic acidosis associated with renal failure. Correction of this metabolic derangement has been shown to improve constitutional growth and improve the sense of well-being in these patients. Patients with glomerular filtration rates less than 40 ml/min/1.73 m^2 should especially be considered for augmentation with stomach.[65] Patients with oliguric or anuric renal failure may also be considered for gastric augmentation. However, special consideration (i.e., H2 antagonists) needs to be given to protect the mucosa and epithelium in these patients until urine is more readily available after renal transplantation to buffer the gastric secretions.

Patients with compromized intestinal length are also potential candidates for gastric augmentation. This patient population would include patients who have short gut secondary to previous intestinal resection, radiation enteritis, cloacal exstrophy, or inflammatory bowel disease. Use of stomach preserves the remaining intestine available for fluid and nutrient absorption, which is critical in this patient population.

Patients prone to fecal incontinence should also be considered for gastrocystoplasty if they require bladder augmentation. Fecal incontinence and/or diarrhea can occur transiently or chronically after bowel resection, especially when the ileocecal valve has been removed from continuity with the gastrointestinal tract. Loss of bowel control has been noted in some patients after ileocystoplasty as well.[65] Patients particularly at risk for this include those with imperforate anus and those with spina bifida who rely on controlled constipation for fecal continence.

Because gastrocystoplasty has been associated with a very low rate of bladder calculus formation, it may also be considered in those patients who require bladder augmentation but are prone to stone formation based on their previous clinical history. This especially holds true for patients prone to infectious stone formation.

These patient populations are most likely to benefit from the advantages that stomach has to offer over other bowel segments. Gastrocystoplasty should be strongly considered in these patients.

CONCLUSIONS

The gastric flap for bladder augmentation or continent reservoir construction has proven to be a valuable technique in certain clinical settings. This is particularly true in complex patients requiring reconstruction who have deficiency of other tissues (i.e., cloacal exstrophy patients, myelodysplastic patients, and patients after radiation therapy). Stomach is remarkably similar to the native bladder and therefore facilitates the construction of tunnels for continent stomas and for ureteral reimplantation. Because of acid excretion, it is very useful in the child with a tendency toward metabolic acidosis. Disadvantages of using stomach must be considered before selecting it for urinary reconstruction. Bladder reconstruction with the use of demucosalized gastric segments and/or composite intestinal components in urinary reconstruction may ultimately alleviate some of these problems in the future.

REFERENCES

1. Ferris, D.O. and Odel, H.M. (1950) Electrolyte pattern of blood after bilateral ureterosigmoidostomy. *Journal of the American Medical Association*, **142**, 634.
2. Bristol, J.B. and Williamson, R.C. (1981) Ureterosigmoidostomy and colon carcinogenesis. *Science*, **214**, 851.
3. Hensle, T. and Dean, G. (1991) Complications of urinary tract reconstruction. *Urologic Clinics of North America,* **18**(4) 755.
4. Sinaiko, E.S. (1956) Artificial bladder from segment of stomach and study of effect of urine on gastric secretion. *Surgery, Gynecology and Obstetrics*, **102**, 433.
5. Leong, C.H. (1972) Gastrocystoplasty in dogs. *Australian and New Zealand Journal of Surgery,* **41**, 272.
6. Rudick, J., Schonholz, S. and Weber, H. (1977) The gastric bladder: a continent reservoir for urinary diversion. *Surgery*, **82**, 1.
7. Piser, J.A., Mitchell, M.E., Kulb, T.B. *et al.* (1987) Gastrocystoplasty and colocystoplasty in canines: the metabolic consequences of acute saline and acid loading. *Journal of Urology,* **138**, 1009.
8. Mitchell, M.E. and Piser, J.A. (1987) Intestinocystoplasty and total bladder replacement in children and young adults: follow-up in 129 cases. *Journal of Urology,* **138**, 579.
9. Dykes, E.H. and Ransley, P.G. (1992) Gastrocystoplasty in children. *British Journal of Urology,* **69**, 91.
10. Leong, C.H. (1988) The use of gastrocystoplasty. *Dialogues in Pediatric Urology*, 2–3.
11. Hull, B.E. and Staehelin, L.A. (1976) Functional significance of the variations in the geometrical organization of tight junction networks. *Journal of Cell Biology*, **68**(3), 688.
12. Mitchell, M.E. and Horowitz, M (1995) The gastric continent urinary reservoir. In *Urinary Diversion, Scientific Foundation and Clinical Practice.*Webster,G.D. and Goldwasser, B. (eds.) Oxford, Isis Medical Media: 185–91.
13. Mitchell, M.E. (1991) Stomach for bladder augmentation and replacement. In *Bladder Reconstruction and Continent Urinary Diversion.* King, L.R., Stone, A.R. and Webster, G.D. (eds.) Chicago, Mosby Year Book: 000–000.
14. Bogaert, G.A., Mevorach, R.A., Kim, J. *et al.* (1995) The physiology of gastrocystoplasty: once a stomach, always a stomach. *Journal of Urology,* **153**, 1977–80.
15. Rink, R.C. and Mitchell, M.E. (1991) Gastrocystoplasty. In *Problems in Urology. Use of Gastrointestinal Segments in Urologic Surgery.* Rowland, G. and Randall G. (guest ed.). Philadelphia, J.B. Lippincott: 213–23.
16. Kennedy, H.A., Adams, M.C., Mitchell, M.E. *et al,* (1988) Chronic renal failure and bladder augmentation: stomach versus sigmoid colon in the canine model. *Journal of Urology,* **140,** 1138.
17. Adams, M.C., Mitchell, M.E. and Rink, R.C. (1988) Gastrocystoplasty: an alternative solution to the problem of urological reconstruction in the severely compromised patient. *Journal of Urology,* **140**, 1152.
18. Ganesan, G.S., Mitchell, M.E., Burns, M.B. *et al.* (1991) Bladder reconstruction using stomach: 73 patients in six years later. (Abstract 158). Presented at American Urological Association Meeting, Washington, DC. *Journal of Urology,* **147**, 253A.
19. Sheldon, C.A., Gilbert, A., Wacksman, J. *et al.* (1995) Gastrocystoplasty: technical and metabolic characteristics of the most versatile childhood bladder augmentation modality. *Journal of Pediatric Surgery,* **30**, 283.
20. Koch, M.O. and McDougall, W.S. (1985) The pathophysiology of hyperchloremic metabolic acidosis after urinary diversion through intestinal segments. *Surgery*, **98**(2), 561.
21. Rink, R.C. and Mitchell, M.E. (1991) Role of enterocystoplasty in reconstructing the neurogenic bladder. In *Problems in Urology*. Gonzaelez, R. (ed.) St Louis, Mosby Yearbook: 192–202.
22. Hendren, W.H. and Hendren, R.B. (1990) Bladder

augmentation: experience with 129 children and young adults. *Journal of Urology,* **144**, 445.

23. Kulb, T.B., Rink, R.C. and Mitchell, M.E. (1986) Gastrocystoplasty in azotemic canines. Presented at North Central Section, American Urological Association Meeting.
24. Klee, L.W., Hoover, D.M., Mitchell, M.E. *et al.* (1990) Long term effects of gastrocystoplasty in rats. *Journal of Urology,* **144**, 1283.
25. Lewis, A.G., Gardner, B., Gilbert, A. *et al.* (1995) Relative microbial resistance of gastric, ileal, and cecal bladder augmentation in the rat. *Journal of Urology,* **154**, 1895.
26. Hollensbe, D.W., Adams, M.C., Rink, R.C. *et al.* (1992) Comparison of various gastrointestinal segments for bladder augmentation. Presented at the National AUA meeting, Washington, DC.
27. Blythe, B., Ewalt, D.H. and Duckett, J.W. (1992) Lithogenic properties of enterocystoplasty. *Journal of Urology,* **148**, 575.
28. Palmer, L.S., Franco, I., Kogan, S.J., *et al.* (1993) Urolithiasis in children following augmentation cystoplasty. *Journal of Urology,* **150**, 726.
29. Garzotto, M.G. and Walker, R.D. (1995) Uric acid stone and gastric bladder augmentation. *Journal of Urology,* **153**, 1976.
30. Adams, M.C., Birhle, R. and Rink, R.C. (1995) The use of stomach in urologic reconstruction. *AUA Update Series,* **XIV**(Lesson 27), 218.
31. Goodwin, W. Personal communication.
32. Ganesan, G.S., Nguyen, D.H., Adams, M.C. *et al.* (1993) Lower urinary tract reconstruction using stomach and artificial urinary sphincter. *Journal of Urology,* **149**, 1107.
33. Atala, A., Bauer, S.B., Hendren, W.H. *et al.* (1993) The effect of gastric augmentation on bladder function. *Journal of Urology,* **149**, 1099.
34. Gosalbez, R. Jr, Woodard, J.R., Broecker, B.H. *et al.* (1992) Urodynamics of gastrocystoplasty and continent gastric reservoirs: a critical review. Presented at the American Academy of Pediatrics, Urology Section Meeting, San Francisco.
35. Ngan, J., Lau, J., Lim, S. *et al.* (1993) Long-term results of antral gastrocystoplasty. *Journal of Urology,* **149**, 731.
36. Rink, R.C., Keating, M.A. and Adams, M.C. (1991) Augmenting the augmented bladder: addressing persistent incontinence. Presented at the American Academy of Pediatrics, Urology Section Meeting, New Orleans, LA.
37. Atala, A., Bauer, S.B. and Hendren, W.H. (1994) Urodynamics of gastrocystoplasty. *Dialogues in Pediatric Urology*, **17**(9), 6–7.
38. Sumfest, J.M. and Mitchell, M.E. (1994) Gastrocystoplasty in children. *European Urology,* **25**, 89.
39. Ueoka, K., Tanikaze, S. and Sugita, Y. (1994) Gastrocystoplasty in pediatric patients. *Nippon Hinyokika Gakkai Zasshi*, **85**(8), 289.
40. Bogaert, G.A., Mevorach, R.A. and Kogan, B.A. (1994) Urodynamic and clinical follow-up of 28 children after gastrocystoplasty. *British Journal of Urology,* **74**, 469.
41. Gosalbez, R. Jr, Woodard, J.R., Broecker, B.H. *et al.* (1993) The use of stomach in pediatric urinary reconstruction. *Journal of Urology,* **150**, 438.
42. Nakagawa, T.A., Gomez, R.J. and Dougan, M.L. (1994) Severe metabolic alkalosis after bladder reconstruction. *Pediatric Emergency Care,* **10**(4), 213.
43. Kinahan, T., Khoury, A.E., McLorie, G.A. *et al.* (1992) Omeprazole in post-gastrocystoplasty metabolic alkalosis and aciduria. *Journal of Urology,* **147**, 435.
44. Mitchell, M.E. (1994) Metabolic complications of the use of stomach. *Dialogues in Pediatric Urology*, **17**(9), 4–5.
45. Schiller, L.R., Walsh, J.H. and Feldman, M. (1980) Distension-induced gastrin release: effects of luminal acidification and intravenous atropine. *Gastroenterology*, **78**, 912.
46. Plawker, M.W., Rabinowitz, S.S, Etwaru, D.J. *et al.* (1995) Hypergastrinemia, dysuria–hematuria and metabolic alkalosis: complications associated with gastrocystoplasty. *Journal of Urology,* **154**(2, Part 1), 546.
47. Nguyen, D.H., Bain, M.A., Salmonson, K.L. *et al.* (1993) The syndrome of dysuria and hematuria in pediatric urinary reconstruction with stomach. *Journal of Urology,* **150**, 707.
48. Festen, H.P., Thijs, J.C. and Lamers, C.B. (1984) Effects of oral omeprazole on serum gastrin and serum pepsinogen I levels. *Gastroenterology*, **87**(5), 1030.
49. Arnold, R. and Koop, H. (1989) Omeprazole: long-term safety. *Digestion*, **44** (Suppl. 1), 77.
50. Muraishi, O., Ikado, S., Yamashita, T. *et al.* (1992)

Gastrocystoplasty in dogs: an ulcerating effect of acid urine. *Journal of Urology,* **147**(1), 242.

51. Castro Diaz, D., Froemming, C., Manivel, J. *et al.* (1992) The influence of urinary diversion on experimental gastrocystoplasty. *Journal of Urology,* **148**(2, Part 2), 571.
52. Muraishi, O., Ogawa, A., Kato, H. *et al.* (1994) Gastrocystoplasty in adults and postoperative aciduria. *Nippon Hinyokika Gakkai Zasshi,* **85**(8), 1263.
53. Reinberg, Y., Manivel, J., Froemming, C. *et al.* (1992) Perforation of the gastric segment of an augmented bladder secondary to peptic ulcer disease. *Journal of Urology,* **148**(2, Part 1), 369.
54. Lau, J., Richter, H. III, Fowler, J. Jr *et al.* (1990) Suppression of canine antral gastrin secretion by urine. *Journal of Urology,* **14**, 402.
55. Ngan, J. and Mitchell, M.E. (1998) Gastrocystoplasty. In *Pediatric Surgery and Urology: Long-term Outcomes.* Philadelphia, W.B. Saunders: 596–603.
56. Gold, B., Bhoopalam, P., Reifen, R. *et al.* (1992) Gastrointestinal complications of gastrocystoplasty. *Archives of Disease in Childhood,* **67**(10), 1272.
57. Merrill, J. and Hampers, C. (1970) Uremia. *New England Journal of Medicine,* **282**, 953.
58. Filmer, R. and Spencer, J. (1990) Malignancies in bladder augmentations and intestinal conduits. *Journal of Urology,* **143**, 671.
59. Little, J., Klee, L., Hoover, D. *et al.* (1994) Long-term histopathological changes observed in rats subjected to augmentation cystoplasty. *Journal of Urology,* **152**, 720.
60. Buson, H., Castro Diaz, D., Manivel, J. *et al.* (1993) The development of tumors in experimental gastrocystoplasty. *Journal of Urology,* **150**(2, Part 2), 730.
61. Spencer, J., Steckel, J., May, M. *et al.* (1993) Histological and bacteriological findings in long-term ileocystoplasty and colocystoplasty in the rat. *Journal of Urology,* **150**, 1321.
62. Bissada, S. and Bissada, N. (1992) Choice of gastroepiploic vessels for gastrocystoplasty. *Journal of Urology,* **148**(1), 101.
63. McLaughlin, K.P., Rink, R.C., Adams, M.C. *et al.* (1995) Stomach in combination with other intestinal segments in pediatric lower urinary tract reconstruction. *Journal of Urology,* **154**(3), 1162.
64. Barone, J and Woodard, J.D. (1994) Patient selection for gastrocystoplasty. *Dialogues in Pediatric Urology,* **17**(9), 5–6.

7

Complications of enterocystoplasty

CLARE E CLOSE

INTRODUCTION

Bladder replacement and augmentation are considered commonplace procedures in adults and children. Enterocystoplasty, first described in 1899, was initially used in cases of urinary tuberculosis, carcinoma of the bladder, and interstitial cystitis.[1] After the popularization of clean intermittent catheterization (CIC) by Lapides in 1972, the use of bladder augmentation expanded to include the primary treatment of small noncompliant bladders and reconstruction after urinary undiversion.[2] With many individuals now over 20 years after augmentation, there are escalating data pertaining to the complications that occur after enterocystoplasty. Although alternative methods of bladder reconstruction without enteric mucosa are being developed, there are thousands of patients who have undergone traditional bladder augmentation who are at risk for both short-term and long-term difficulties that arise when full-thickness enteric segments are added to the urinary tract. The urologic surgeon must remain vigilant to these patients and their potential complications.

METABOLIC AND ELECTROLYTE DISORDERS

Urinary diversion by ureterosigmoidostomy provided the first data regarding metabolic changes and electrolyte disorders that arise when gut segments are placed in the urinary tract. Metabolic acidosis and hyperchloremia developed in 80% of 141 patients in this first series reported by Ferris and Odell.[3] When ileal or colonic segments are used in the urinary tract, the bowel mucosa continues its normal physiologic function and acts as an absorptive surface for urine. Ion absorption and the subsequent development of metabolic abnormality are affected by the type of gut segment used, and the amount of absorptive surface exposed to urine. Electrolytes move across and between the gut mucosal cells by both active and passive transport systems. Chloride and ammonium are selectively reabsorbed from the urine, resulting in hyperchloremic metabolic acidosis.[4] Water moves between the cell junctions according to an osmotic gradient, affected by the tightness of the cell junctions. Moving distally down the bowel segments, the cell junctions allow less and less water loss, such that the colon is relatively impermeable to water. In contrast, the loose cell junctions of the jejunum allow massive water loss, contributing to the serious metabolic complications demonstrated in patients with jejunal conduits.

Early reports of metabolic complications after enterocystoplasty implicated pre-existing renal insufficiency.[5] In a large series of pediatric and adult patients followed long term after augmentation with ileum, colon, cecum, or tubular sigmoid, Mitchell and Piser reported mild hyperchloremia developing in all groups regardless of type of bowel segment used. Acidosis, however, developed only in those patients with renal insufficiency.[6]

In a prospective study of 48 pediatric and adult enterocystoplasty patients, Nurse and Mundy measured electolyte absorption in the augmented bladders after the intravenous administration of radiolabelled isotopes.[7] They reported hyperchloremia in 26% of patients with ileocystoplasties and in 50% of patients with ileocecal bladder substitution. All patients had abnormal blood gases, with the majority demonstrating metabolic acidosis with respiratory compensation. There was a trend toward decreased reabsorption with time after surgery in patients who had undergone reconstruction with ileum, but not in patients with ileocecal segments. The authors suggest that this may reflect villous atrophy in the ileal segment, as previously described in ileal conduits and continent reservoirs.[8,9] The data are, however, not serial measurements on the same patient and no conclusion regarding the natural history of the gut mucosa in each patient can be reached from this study. Although increased time of exposure of gut mucosa to urine would seem to increase the risk for metabolic changes, Nurse and Mundy[7] found that augmentation cystoplasties had no greater risk of metabolic abnormality than that seen with bowel conduits that continuously drain.

STONES

Urinary tract calculi are a potentially serious complication of enterocystoplasty. Pyelonephritis, multiple operations, and even death are reported in two large series addressing urolithiasis after bladder augmentation in children.[10,11] Adult series of enterocystoplasty and bladder substitution have either not mentioned calculi as a complication or have found a low incidence in their patient population.[12,13] The reported incidence of stone formation after augmentation in children ranges widely from 3% to 52%.[6,10,11,14] Mitchell and Piser followed 129 patients with a mean age of 13.4 years after urinary tract reconstruction with bowel. They reported stones in only 3% of these patients after a mean 44-month follow-up.[6] In a large series of bladder augmentation in children and young adults, Hendren and Hendren reported stones as their most common postoperative complication, occurring in 23 of 129 patients (18%). However, almost 75% of the stones occurred after cecal cystoplasty and half of the stones occurred on staples of the antireflux nipple. Their stone incidences following sigmoid or ileal augmentation were 6% and 10% respectively.[14] A higher incidence was reported by Blyth *et al.*, who found urinary tract calculi in 30% of 87 children with bladder augmentation or substitution. In contrast to the patient populations of Mitchell and Hendren,[6,14] however, the majority of Blyth's patients had undergone sigmoid colocystoplasty and almost half emptied through a Mitrofanoff catheterisable conduit.[10] Palmer *et al.*[11] reported an incidence of 52% in 48 augmented patients under the age of 25 years. The median time to stone formation was 2 years or less in both series, with a range from 2 to 72 months. Stone recurrence appears common, with these authors reporting an incidence of 20%.

A metabolic etiology for urolithiasis after augmentation seems unlikely. Palmer *et al.*[11] analysed 24-hour urines in their stone-formers and found hypocitraturia to be the only abnormality. The children were treated with oral potassium citrate and no recurrence of urolithiasis was noted. Postaugmentation, upper tract stones occurred in three of 26 stone-formers (12%), with no patients in the series admitting to preaugmentation urolithiasis.[11] Blyth *et al.* reported upper tract stones in 15% of their patients prior to augmentation but did not find upper tract recurrence after augmentation.[10]

Metal surgical staples have been implicated in stone formation in continent urinary reservoirs and augmented bladders.[14,15] Palmer *et al.* found an association between absorbable staple use and stone formation. They found absorbable staple 'ghosts' within bladder calculi as well as calculi attached to metal staples.[11] Blyth *et al.* reported one calculus on a permanent bladder neck suture, but no stones associated with absorbable suture closure of the bladder.[10]

Persistent bacteruria is a leading cause of stone formation after enterocystoplasty. Bladder stone composition after augmentation with bowel is predominantly apatite, struvite and ammonium urate. Infection with urease-splitting organisms causes alkaline urine and an increased concentration of phosphate ion, with subsequent formation of calcium phosphate and struvite stones. Struvite was the major component in ileocystoplasty stones, whereas ileocecocystoplasties had the highest composition of ammonium urate stones in the series reported by Blyth *et al.*.[10]

Although infection may be the major etiologic factor in stone formation, urine stasis predisposes many patients to infection and subsequent stones. Urine is commonly retained in the augmented bladder due to an abnormal bladder contour and inefficient drainage. Poor sensation in the augmented bladder and increased bladder capacity result in less frequent intermittent catheterization in some patients. The data of Blyth *et al.* suggest that Mitrofanoff drainage may be a further risk factor for stone formation, with one-third of their reported stone patients emptying via an appendicovesicostomy.[10] The use of small drainage catheters and the dependent position of the bladder relative to the catheterisable channel may result in poor drainage of material particulates.

Retention of mucus in the augmented bladder is common and appears to contribute to infection and stone formation in some patients. Khoury *et al.* evaluated the mucus and urine of stone-formers and nonstone-formers.[16] Both groups demonstrated hypocitraturia. Notably, the mucus of the stone-formers was significantly higher in calcium, phosphate, and magnesium when compared to that of the nonstone-formers. Furthermore, nine of ten stones examined had fluid centers containing high concentrations of calcium, phosphate, and magnesium, suggesting mucus as the nidus. The calcium:phosphate ratio was a positive predictor of stone formation in these patients.

Gastrocystoplasty affords resistance to stone formation due to the acidic milieu of the gastric augmentation and the character of the mucus. Garzotto and Walker[17] report one case of a pure uric acid bladder stone diagnosed seven months after gastrocystoplasty. This patient had mild hypercalcuria and hypercalcemia demonstrated on a 24-hour urine collection. They hypothesize that acidic gastrocystoplasty urine predisposed the patient to stone formation, as uric acid crystalizes below its pKa of 5.75.

Attention to stone prevention is necessary in patients with traditional enteric bladder augmentation. Antibiotic prophylaxis against infection is not recommended except in patients with vesicoureteral reflux. Inhibition of the urease reaction by acetohydroxamic acid therapy has not yet been adequately tested.[10] Diligent catheterization with thorough bladder emptying is essential for the prevention of primary and recurrent stones. If initial bladder stones are secondary to poor bladder emptying or mucus retention, then stones are likely to recur unless bladder management is changed. Khoury *et al.* recommend prophylactic irrigations of the augmented bladders to break-up entrapped mucus and thoroughly flush the bladder. Daily irrigation with 300 cm^3 of tap water was shown to decrease the incidence of stone formation in children with bladder augmentation.[16]

The management of a stone burden can utilize all endoscopic and open procedures used for urolithiasis. For large bladder stones, open cystolithopaxy is often the treatment of choice.[10] Smaller stones may be removed endoscopically, although the abnormal contour of augmented bladders as well as the difficulties of working through the reconstructed bladder neck or Mitrofanoff channel make endoscopic treatment difficult. Palmer *et al.* used cystoscopic treatment in 18 of 25 cases (72%) but did not report the number of simple extractions versus electrohydraulic lithotripsy.[11] If extracorporeal shockwave lithotripsy or electrohydraulic lithotripsy is utilized, all stone fragments must be removed, a process which is difficult in these bladders. Alternative treatment for bladder lithiasis includes intravesical dissolution. Blyth *et al.* attempted treatment with intravesical hemiacidrin and reported a stone-free rate of 24% at 1 year.[10] However, resorbtion of salts, particularly magnesium, may be a problem with this method of treatment.

PERFORATION

Although considered a rare complication, bladder perforation after augmentation is a life-threatening complication. Delay in diagnosis due to lack of normal sensation in many patients undergoing enterocystoplasty, combined with lack of suspicion on the part of managing physicians, has resulted in death in some patients.[18,19]

The etiology of bladder perforation remains ambiguous. The proposed mechanisms of perforation include catheter trauma, chronic infection, avulsion of adhesions, ischemia, and chronic overdistension with increased intravesical pressure. In the 90 pediatric perforations reported in the literature since 1977, 78 (87%) occurred in patients with a neurogenic bladder.[20] Eighty-seven percent of the perforations occurred in patients on intermittent catheterization, with failure to catheterize documented in almost 20%. These patients with poor sensation and competent bladder necks are at high risk for developing asymptomatic overdistension of the augmented bladder.

Bladder perforation has been reported in all enteric segments, with an incidence between 5% and 7% reported in the largest series.[18,21] Data concerning the risk for rupture in each type of augmentation are conflicting. Bauer *et al.* found the highest incidence of perforation after ileocystoplasty, whereas Pope *et al.* found sigmoid augmentation to have the greatest rate of perforation.[18,21] Variables such as the use of tubularized segments and the use of procedures to increase bladder outlet resistance make it difficult to reach conclusions of risk for each bowel segment.

The pathologic changes in the augmented bladder that lead to perforation remain ill-defined. Approximately half of the perforation cases in the literature were surgically explored. Of these cases, 72% demonstrated rupture through the bowel segment, while the remainder ruptured through the anastomotic zone. In the series by Bauer *et al.*, 80% of the perforations at the anastomotic site are an early occurrence, reported at a mean of less than 4 months after augmentation.[18] The ruptures happened in the junctional zone between gut and bladder segments as well as at the bowel to bowel anastomosis of the detubularized reconfigured enteric segment. In an experimental model of bladder rupture in rats, Chancellor *et al.* found a similar pattern in site of rupture after ileocystoplasty. Sixty-four percent of the animal bladders ruptured through the dome of the ileal segment, while the remainder perforated through the anastomotic zone between bowel and bladder.[22]

The literature contains only scattered histologic data from material taken at the time of surgical exploration. Histopathologic analysis of the sites of rupture suggest ischemia as a plausible etiology of perforation in some cases. Bauer *et al.* described thinning of the enteric segment with fibrotic replacement of the muscularis.[18] Crane *et al.* found changes in the perforated bowel wall consistent with long-standing vascular compromise, including myofiber atrophy, intravascular thrombi, and hemosiderin-filled macrophages.[23]

Crane *et al.* present a cogent hypothesis for the mechanism by which chronic overdistension leads to perforation.[23] Ischemic damage from vascular compromise in the bowel wall can result from increased wall tension secondary to chronic distension and increased intralumenal pressure.[24,25] According to the law of Laplace, in any sphere, wall tension increases directly as intraluminal pressure and/or sphere radius increases.[26] Wall tension is thus increased as the bladder is distended, even though the intravesical pressure remains low. Because of its spherical shape, the bladder's radius after augmentation is typically greatest through the augmentation segment. This will be the area of highest wall tension and, as demonstrated in the existing clinical reports, the site at highest risk for rupture. If maximum tolerated wall tension in the augmented bladder is reached at pressures below leak-point pressure, the augmentation segment will perforate. Accordingly, conditions that increase leak-point pressure, such as the presence of an artificial urinary sphincter, bladder neck reconstruction, or urethral mucus plugging, further increase the danger of perforation. As evidenced in the published studies, the risk of perforation is increased with concomitant procedures to increase bladder neck resistance. The attempt to make patients totally dry with bladder augmentation combined with bladder neck procedures is reported in over 50% of the perforation patients.[21]

In a case of a defunctionalized gastrocystoplasty, Reinberg *et al.* described perforation through a site of peptic ulceration. Histopathologic analysis of this specimen demonstrated not only ischemic changes but also metaplasia of the incorporate gastric mucosa.[27] These authors hypothesize that mucosal ischemia and the loss of the protective effect of alkaline urine in the bladder resulted in an increased susceptibility to ulceration and subsequent perforation after gastrocystoplasty.

Patients with bladder perforation present with a variety of signs and symptoms ranging from silent urinoma to florid sepsis and shock.[18,20] Abdominal pain or pain radiating to the shoulder is common, secondary to peritoneal irritation, but may be absent in the myelomeningocele patients with decreased abdominal sensation. Silent or painless presentation may be due to loculation of the leak and may explain why some patients have been managed successfully with percutaneous drainage only.[20] The cystogram has been the most commonly used diagnostic tool for perforation, with a 20% false-negative rate calculated from the published reports.[21] A combined cystogram and CT scan is thought to improve the accuracy of either study. A high index of suspicion for perforation in any augmentation patient should be maintained and immediate surgical exploration initiated in gravely ill patients. Delay in diagnosis and failure to resuscitate the patient adequately can lead to a rapid downhill course and death.[18,19]

NEOPLASTIC PROGRESSION

Twenty years after the early augmentation cystoplasties were performed, Smith and Hardy reported the first tumor in an augmented bladder.[28] This was a poorly differentiated transitional cell carcinoma with squamous elements that developed on the ileal segment near the ileovesical junction 17 years after augmentation. Since this report, 15 additional cases have been reported.[29] The 16 tumors include nine adenocarcinomas, three transitional cell carcinomas, one oat cell carcinoma, one sarcoma, one signet ring cell carcinoma, and one case of a synchronous signet ring cell carcinoma and sarcoma. Thirteen of the 16 patients (81%) had a history of tuberculosis or chronic cystitis prior to augmentation. The consequences of the tumor development were grave, with at least one-third of the patients dying from the disease. In 80% of the patients the tumor developed near the junctional zone between the bowel segment and the native bladder. Bowel segments involved include ileum, jejunum, and colon.

To date, no cases have been reported in patients after gastrocystoplasty. However, with the hundreds of children who have undergone gastrocystoplasty there is growing concern for the possibility of neoplasia arising in these bladders.

Prognostication about the potential for tumorigenesis after gastrocystoplasty stems from long-term animal models. Several studies of gastric augmentation in the rat have demonstrated proliferative lesions in the anastomotic zone between the gastric wedge and the native bladder.[30–2] Buson *et al.* found papillary hyperplasia in over 50% of animals surviving 1 year after gastrocystoplasty.[30] They interpret these as non-neoplastic and not premalignant. The nomenclature used to describe proliferative lesions is, however, not uniform and can lead to varying conclusions regarding the malignant potential of the lesions. Other authors report transitional cell metaplasia or hyperplasia in all animals surviving 1 to 2 years after gastrocystoplasty.[31,32] Klee *et al.* identified an apparent squamous carcinoma in one bladder with a papilloma. Using flow cytometric analysis of cell cycle profiles, Close *et al.* found near-diploid DNA aneuploidy in the proliferative lesions of one of 12 experimental animals.[32]

Although hyperplasia can occur normally during healing of a bowel anastomosis, there is evidence that it can predispose the intestinal tract to neoplasm. Animal experiments demonstrate that in bowel exposed to a known carcinogen, the potential for tumor development is significantly higher in the anastomotic line than elsewhere on the mucosal surface. Furthermore, the tumorigenic risk persists beyond the healing phase. It may be that carcinogens act selectively on the rapidly dividing cells at the anastomosis. Crypt cell proliferation in the anastomotic line increases significantly for at least 3 months after the anastomosis. The increased susceptibility of the anastomotic zone cells to carcinogenesis persists through the time of increased rate of cell proliferation and suggests that even when healed, the anastomoses remain the preferential site for neoplastic change.[33] Close *et al.* found a junctional zone cell turnover rate ten times that of the control transitional cell epithelium after long-term gastrocystoplasty in Long–Evans rats.[32] If rapidly dividing cells are at increased risk for carcinogenesis, then these data suggest an increased potential for neoplasm in the gastrocystoplasty anastomotic line.

There are clinical data suggesting increased susceptibility to tumorigenesis during the healing phase after bowel to urinary tract anastomosis in humans. Carcinomas have developed in ureterosigmoidostomy patients with bowel segments exposed to the urinary stream for less than 1 year.[34] These patients had ureteral stumps retained in the colon segments and therefore a persistence of the susceptible anastomotic zone, albeit without any further exposure to possible urinary carcinogens.

Anastomoses between bladder and enteric segments may be at higher risk for carcinogenesis than the junctional zone between bowel to bowel anastomoses. In animal studies of ureterosigmoidostomy modified by bowel segment interposition between sigmoid and bladder, tumors developed at the bowel to bladder anastomosis rather than at the bowel to sigmoid anastomosis which was in contact with the fecal and urinary stream.[35] There are increasing data supporting the theory that foreign tissue stroma induces epithelial changes in a variety of organs.[36,37] Two-way interaction between the epithelium and stroma has also been demonstrated in the developing bladder.[38] Normal epithelial development and epithelial tumorigenesis have been found to be mediated by epithelial–mesenchyme interactions in the prostate.[39] Tumor development after bladder augmentation with full-thickness bowel segments may be secondary to such interaction in the anastomotic zone.

The contribution of bacterial infection and possible urinary carcinogens to neoplastic development in the anastomosis remains unclear. Urine nitrites, formed by gram-negative bacteria by the reduction of normally occurring urinary nitrates, are implicated in tumorigenesis in ureterosigmoidostomies and urinary conduits.[40] The reduced nitrates are further catalyzed to nitrosamines which are mutagenic.[41] This same mechanism could be acting in the augmented bladder, where bacterial colonization is common. The majority of augmented patients practice CIC and are not treated for bacteruria unless they are symptomatic or have associated vesicoureteral reflux. Whether or not this is a major risk factor for neoplastic development is still unknown.

UNIQUE COMPLICATIONS OF GASTROCYSTOPLASTY

Hypochloremic metabolic alkalosis

Stomach mucosal segments placed into the urinary tract retain the ability to secrete hydrogen ions. These ions are produced intracellularly from carbonic acid with the generation of bicarbonate ion that is then secreted systemically. The parietal cells responsible for hydrochloric acid secretion are found in the body and fundus of the bladder and are always present in the traditional gastric augmentation wedge. Metabolic abnormality after gastrocystoplasty occurs less frequently than after augmentation with bowel segments. Several authors have, however, reported severe hyponatremic hypochloremic metabolic alkalosis after gastrocystoplasty.[42–4] Ganesan *et al.* described the abnormality in nine of 73 patients (12%), with one patient requiring take-down of the gastric segment.[44]

Excess systemic bicarbonate is typically excreted by the kidneys into urine and theoretically neutralizes acidic urine. Early reports of metabolic complications after gastrocystoplasty occurred in renal failure patients, leading to speculation that impaired renal excretion of bicarbonate was the cause of metabolic alkalosis.[45,46] Subsequent series have described serious postgastrocystoplasty metabolic alkalosis in patients with normal renal function.[43,47] These patients experienced hypochloremia and hypokalemia secondary to vomiting and hydrochloric acid loss from the stomach flap. With potassium depletion, renal bicarbonate reabsorption can be increased, perpetuating the alkalosis that began with acid loss.

Hypergastrinemia

Several authors have reported hypergastrinemia in patients with metabolic alkalosis.[43,46,47] In the in-situ stomach, distension and increased intraluminal pH stimulate gastrin secretion from the antral G cells. Hydrochloric acid is then secreted by parietal cells in response to circulating gastrin. Augmentation using the antrum of the stomach might then be expected to result in increased acid secretion into the urine with bladder distension. The experimental and clinical data conflict in this regard. Tiffany *et al.* described severe hypergastrinemia after antral gastrocystoplasty in dogs.[48] Lim *et al.*, however, reported 13 patients with an antral gastrocystoplasty and normal gastrin levels.[49] If incomplete denervation of the stomach flap occurs with mobilization, then theoretically, retained G cells in the augmentation flap would secrete gastrin in response to bladder stretch. Retained antrum in the gastrocystoplasty wedge is usually avoided when the gastrocystoplasty wedge popularized by Adams, Mitchell *et al.* is used as it avoids the lesser curve of the stomach.[45] However, variable distribution of G cells is possible and selection of the wedge is sometimes more dependent on the distribution of flap feeding vessels than the exact location on the stomach body. Again, there are conflicting data regarding the role of gastrin in postgastrocystoplasty aciduria when the augmentation flap is harvested from the body of the stomach. Muraishi *et al.* found elevated serum gastrin levels 3 months after gastrocystoplasty in dogs, but no persistence of hypergastrinemia. These animals did develop mucosal erosions and ulceration in the augmented native bladder, but no similar changes in the gastric mucosa.[50] In a prospective study of gastrocystoplasties from the body of the stomach, Bogaert *et al.* investigated gastrin secretion in response to bladder and stomach distension.[51] They found an increase in serum gastrin after stomach distension with food, but no increase in acid secretion or serum gastrin with bladder distension. Urinary pH fell and titratable acids increased in parallel to serum gastrin increase. These data support the theory that gastrin secretion from in-situ stomach acts on gastrocystoplasty parietal cells to produce acid.

Factors other than gastrin stimulation have been implicated in increased acid production by the augmentation flap. Dykes and Ransley suggest that the size of the gastric flap is a factor in the amount of acid produced. Additionally, they report one child on prednisone therapy after renal transplantation with increased aciduria.[52]

Hematuria–dysuria syndrome

Hematuria–dysuria syndrome is a complication unique to bladder augmentation with full-thickness stomach flaps. Strictly, it is defined as: dysuria and hematuria in the absence of infection, skin irritation or excoriation, and suprapubic or perineal pain. Typically, the symptoms are mild and do not require medication; the problem can be severe enough to require take-down of the gastric segment.[46] Nguyen *et al.*[53] first named the syndrome in 1993, although other authors had previously described the same constellation of symptoms.[46,52]

Since these early reports, several authors have speculated on the possible etiology and there are conflicting views on the presence of aciduria and elevated gastrin levels in the syndrome: Dykes and Ransley reported gross hematuria and severe dysuria after gastrocystoplasty in two of eight children with compromized renal function. One of these patients demonstrated normal serum chloride and gastrin levels, but elevated levels of urinary titratable acids. Both patients improved with oral omeprazole or H-2 receptor blockers.[52] In the large series reported by Nguyen *et al.* there was no difference between the preprandial and postprandial urine pH levels.[53] Plawker *et al.* found refractory metabolic alkalosis associated with hematuria and dysuria in a patient with renal insufficiency. Their patient had severe hypergastrinemia but, interestingly, alkaline urine.[47] Intravesical pH can, however, be significantly lower than the pH of voided urine and this fact may account for the difference in findings reported by the various authors.[52]

Other factors leading to the hematuria–dysuria syndrome have been suggested; one child's symptoms resolved after starting intermittent catheterization, suggesting that Valsava voiding and incomplete emptying may exacerbate the problem.[51]

Oliguria could be expected to exacerbate any irritative process due to the long exposure of the mucosa to urine between infrequent voids. In their original series, Nguyen *et al.* found that symptoms occurred more frequently in patients with renal insufficiency.[53] Similarly, Sheldon *et al.* reported hematuria–dysuria in an end-stage renal failure patient which resolved with transplantation.[54] Urinary incontinence is another risk factor, occurring in up to 60% of patients with the syndrome.[53] The child with a sensate perineum who dribbles urine is logically at higher risk for dysuria than the continent child or the child with decreased sensation.

Recently, Celayir *et al.* suggested an infectious etiology for the syndrome of hematuria and dysuria. *Heliobacter pylori* seropositivity was found in four of nine patients (44%) studied retrospectively after gastrocystoplasty. All had symptoms of hematuria and dysuria syndrome and one of the four had positive *Heliobacter pylori* cultured from an augmentation biopsy.[55] Additional prospective investigation is needed to clarify the role of infection in this unique complication.

REFERENCES

1. Mikuliez, J. (1899) Zur operation der Angeborenen Blasenspalte. *Zentralblatt für Chirurgie,* **26,** 641–3.
2. Lapides, J., Diokno, A.C., Silber, S.J. *et al.* (1972) Clean intermittent self-catheterization in the treatment of urinary tract disease. *Journal of Urology,* **107,** 458–61.
3. Ferris, D.O. and Odell, H.M. (1950) Electrolyte pattern of the blood after bilateral ureterosigmoidostomy. *Journal of the American Medical Association,* **142,** 634–40.
4. McDougal, W.S. (1992) Metabolic complication of urinary intestinal diversion. *Journal of Urology,* **147,** 1199–208.
5. Kass, E.J. and Koff, S.A. (1983) Bladder augmentation in the pediatric neuropathic bladder. *Journal of Urology,* **129,** 552–5.
6. Mitchell, M.E. and Piser, J.A. (1987) Intestinocystoplasty and total bladder replacement in children and young adults: follow-up in 129 cases. *Journal of Urology,* **138,** 579–84.
7. Nurse, D.E. and Mundy, A.R. (1989) Metabolic complications of cystoplasty. *British Journal of Urology,* **63,** 165–70.
8. Deane, A.M., Woodhouse, C.R.J. and Parkinson, M.C. (1984) Histologic changes in ileal conduits. *Journal of Urology,* **132,** 1108–11.
9. Hansson, H-A., Kock, N.G., Norlen, L. *et al.* (1978) Morphologic observations in pedicled ileal grafts used for construction of continent reservoirs for urine. *Scandanavian Journal of Urology and Nephrology,* Suppl. **49**, chapter VI, pp.49.
10. Blyth, B., Ewalt, D.H,, Duckett, J.W. and Snyder, H.M III. (1992) Lithogenic properties of enterocystoplasty. *Journal of Urology,* **148,** 575–7.
11. Palmer, L.S., Franco, I., Kogen, S.J. *et al.* (1993) Urolithiasis in children following augmentation cystoplasty. *Journal of Urology,* **150,** 726–9.
12. Smith, R.B., Van Cangh, P., Skinner, D.G. *et al.* (1977) Augmentation enterocystoplasty: a critical review. *Journal of Urology,* **118,** 35–9.
13. Lilien, O.M. and Camey, M. (1984) Twenty-five year experience with replacement of the human bladder (Camey procedure). *Journal of Urology,* **132,** 886–91.
14. Hendren, W.H. and Hendren, R.B. (1990) Bladder augmentation: experience with 129 children and young adults. *Journal of Urology,* **144,** 445–53.
15. Ginsberg, D., Huffman, J.L., Lieskovsky, G. *et al.* (1991) Urinary tract stones: a complication of the Kock pouch continent urinary diversion. *Journal of Urology,* **145,** 956–9.
16. Khoury, A.E., Salomon, M., Jayanthi, R. *et al.* (1997) The role of urinary constituents and intestinal mucus in lithogenesis following augmentation cystoplasty. Presented at the European Society of Paediatric Urology, 8th Annual Meeting, Rome, April 3–5, Abstract 72.
17. Garzotto, M.G. and Walker, R.D. III (1976) Uric acid stone and gastric bladder augmentation. *Journal of Urology,* **153**.
18. Bauer, S.B., Hendren, W.H., Kozakewich, H. *et al.* (1992) Perforation of the augmented bladder. *Journal of Urology,* **148,** 699–703.
19. Rushton, H.G., Woodard, J.R., Parrot, T.S. *et al.* (1988) Delayed bladder rupture after augmentation enterocystoplasty. *Journal of Urology,* **140,** 344–6.
20. Close, C.E., Dewan, P.A., Ashwood, P.A. *et al.*

(2000) Bladder perforation after enterocystoplasty: a multicenter report and literature review. *British Journal of Urology International* (submitted).

21. Pope, J.C.IV, Casale, A.J., Adams, M.C. *et al.* (1997) Spontaneous perforation of the augmented bladder: from silence to chaos. *Journal of Urology,* **158,** 2A.
22. Chancellor, M.B., Rivas, D.A. and Bourgeois, I.M. (1996) Laplace's law and the risks and prevention of bladder rupture after enterocystoplasty and bladder autoaugmentation. *Neurourology Urodynamics*, **15,** 223–33.
23. Crane, J.M., Schertz, H.S., Billman, G.F. *et al.* (1991) Ischemic necrosis: a hypothesis to explain the pathogenesis of spontaneously ruptured enterocystoplasty. *Journal of Urology,* **146,** 141–4.
24. Saegesser, F. and Sandblom, P. (1975) Ischemic lesions of the distended colon: a complication of obstructive colorectal cancer. *American Journal of Surgery,* **129,** 309–15.
25. Essig, K.A., Sheldon, C.A., Brandt, M.T. *et al.* (1991) Elevated intravesical pressure causes arterial hypoperfusion in canine colocystoplasty: A flourometric assessment. *Journal of Urology,* **146,** 551–3.
26. Stilwel, G.K. (1973) The law of Laplace. Some clinical applications. *Mayo Clinic Proceedings*, **48,** 863–9.
27. Reinberg, Y., Manivel, J.C., Froemming, C. *et al.* (1992) Perforation of the gastric segment of an augmented bladder secondary to peptic ulcer disease. *Journal of Urology,* **148,** 369–71.
28. Smith, P. and Hardy, G.J. (1971) Carcinoma occurring as a late complication of ileocystoplasty. *British Journal of Urology,* **43,** 576–9.
29. Fernandez-Arjona, M., Herrero, L., Romero, J. *et al.* (1996) Synchronous signet ring cell carcinoma and squamous cell carcinoma arising in an augmented ileocystoplasty. Case report and review of the literature. *European Urology*, **29,** 125–8.
30. Buson, H., Diaz, D.C., Manivel, J.C. *et al.* (1993) The development of tumors in experimental gastroenterocystoplasty. *Journal of Urology*, **150,** 730–3.
31. Klee, L.W., Hoover, D.M., Mitchell, M.E. *et al.* (1990) Long term effects of gastrocystoplasty in rats. *Journal of Urology*, **144,** 1283–7.
32. Close, C.E., Tekgul, S., Ganesan, G.S. *et al.* (1995) Flow cytometric analysis of proliferative lesions at the gastrocystoplasty anastomosis. Presented at the American Academy of Pediatrics Annual Meeting, San Francisco, California, October 1995.
33. Roe, R., Fermor, B. and Williamson, R.C.N. (1987) Proliferative instability and experimental carcinogenesis at colonic anastomoses. *Gut,* **28,** 808–15.
34. Schipper, H. and Decter, A. (1981) Carcinoma of the colon arising at ureteral implant sites despite early external diversion. *Cancer*, **47,** 2062–5.
35. Shands, C., McDougal, W.S. and Wright, E.P. (1989) Prevention of cancer at the urothelial enteric anastomotic line. *Journal of Urology,* **141,** 178–81.
36. Cunha, G.R. and Young, P. (1992) Developmental response of adult mammary epithelial cells to various fetal and neonatal mesenchymes. *Epithelial Cell Biology,* **1,** 105–18.
37. Donjacour, A.A. and Cunha, G.R. (1995) Induction of prostatic morphology and secretion in urothelium by seminal vesicle mesenchyme. *Development*, **121,** 2199–207.
38. Baskin, L.S. and Hayward, S.W. (1996) Role of mesenchymal–epithelial interactions in bladder development. *Journal of Urology,* **156,** 1820–7.
39. Cunha, G.R. and Hayward, S.W. (1996) Smooth muscle–epithelial interactions in normal and neoplastic prostatic development. *Acta Anatomica,* **155,** 63–72.
40. Stewart, M. (1986) Urinary diversion and bowel cancer. *Annals of the Royal College of Surgeons of England*, **68,** 98–102.
41. Shank, R.C. (1975) Toxicology of N-nitrosocompounds. *Toxicology and Applied Pharmacology*, **31,** 361–8.
42. Bogaert, G.A., Mevorach, R.A. and Kogan, B.A. (1994) Urodynamic and clinical follow-up of 28 children after gastrocystoplasty. *British Journal of Urology,* **74,** 469–75.
43. Gosalbez, R.J., Woodard, J.R., Broecker, B.H. *et al.* (1993) Metabolic complications of the use of stomach for urinary reconstruction. *Journal of Urology,* **150,** 710–12.
44. Ganesan, G.S., Mitchell, M.E., Nguyen, D.H. *et al.* (1992) Bladder reconstruction using stomach: 73 patients and 6 years later. *Journal of Urology,* **147,** 253A.
45. Adams, M.C., Mitchell, M.E. and Rink, R.C. (1988)

Gastrocystoplasty: an alternative solution to the problem of urological reconstruction in the severely compromised patient. *Journal of Urology,* **140,** 1152–6.

46. Kinahan, T.J., Khoury, A.E., McLorie, G.A. *et al.* (1992) Omeprazol in post-gastrocystoplasty metabolic alkalosis and aciduria. *Journal of Urology,* **147,** 435–7.
47. Plawker, M.C., Rabinowitz, S.S., Etwaru, D.J. *et al.* (1995) Hypergastrinemia, dysuria-hematuria and metabolic acidosis: complications associated with gastrocystoplasty. *Journal of Urology,* **154,** 546–9.
48. Tiffany, P., Vaughan, E.D. Jr, Marion, D. *et al.* (1986) Hypergastrinemia following antral gastrocystoplasty. *Journal of Urology,* **136,** 692–5.
49. Lim, S.T.K., Lam, S.K., Lee, N.W. *et al.* (1983) Effects of gastrocystoplasty on serum gastrin levels and gastric acid secretion. *British Journal of Urology,* **70,** 275–7.
50. Muraishi, O., Ikado, S., Yamashita, T. *et al.* (1992) Gastrocystoplasty in dogs: an ulcerating effect of acid urine. *Journal of Urology,* **147,** 242–5.
51. Bogaert, G.A., Mevorach, R.A., Kim, J. *et al.* (1995) The physiology of gastrocystoplasty: once a stomach, always a stomach. *Journal of Urology,* **153,** 1977–80.
52. Dykes, E.H. and Ransley, P.G. (1992) Gastrocystoplasty in children. *British Journal of Urology,* **69,** 91–5.
53. Nguyen, D.H., Bain, M.A., Salmonson, K.L. *et al.* (1993) The syndrome of dysuria and hematuria in pediatric urinary reconstruction with stomach. *Journal of Urology,* **150,** 707–9.
54. Sheldon, C.A., Gilbert, A., Wacksman, J., Lewis, A.G. (1995) Gastroplasty: technical and metabolic characteristics of the most versatile childhood bladder augmentation modality. *Journal of Pediatric Surgery,* **30**, 283–8.
55. Celayir, S., Buyukunal, S.N.C. and Suha, G. (1997) The hidden risk of *Heliobacter pylori* infection in paediatric patients with gastric augmentation. Presented at the European Society of Paediatric Urology, 8th Annual Meeting, Rome, April 3–5.

8

Ureterocystoplasty

PADDY DEWAN AND GORDON A MCLORIE

INTRODUCTION

For almost a century, surgeons dealing with bladder dysfunction have recognized the need to enlarge the urinary bladder in certain highly selected instances. The indications for these procedures include a variety of conditions which have, as a common theme, a low bladder capacity, poor compliance, and raised intravesical pressure, which results in urinary incontinence, abdominal pain, recurrent urinary tract infections, vesicoureteral reflux, and in the worst cases, renal parenchyma injury.[1] A perfect and consistent solution for these problems continues to elude us. Conservative medical therapy includes the administration of parasympatholitic drugs (administered both orally and intravesically), intermittent catheterization, bowel management, and prevention of urinary tract infection. However, the results of medical regimens have for the most part been imperfect.

The clinical problems that result from a dysfunctional bladder lead to diverse consequences which often involve either ureterovesical reflux or ureterovesical obstruction. The underlying diagnoses include posterior urethral obstruction,[2–6] bladder exstrophy,[7] neuropathic bladders,[3,5–7] ureteric duplication with reflux,[3,8] and end-stage renal disease,[9] all of which are not infrequently associated with a poorly functioning kidney with a massively dilated refluxing ureter. This has been described as a 'pop-off' or VURD (*v*esico*u*reteric *r*eflux and *d*ysplasia) syndrome,[10] in which unilateral vesicoureteric reflux appears to allow the ipsilateral ureter and its pelvicalyceal system to act as an expansive reservoir, thus preventing contralateral vesicoureteric reflux and renal damage by lowering the bladder pressure.[11] Occasionally, the dilated, poorly functioning system leads to persistent urinary tract infections, suggesting the need for a nephroureterectomy. However, the subsequent removal of the refluxing unit may lead to deterioration in function of the remaining kidney, or of a transplant kidney if both native kidneys have already failed.

Experience with augmentation has most commonly involved the use of ileum, colon, and stomach and has led to an increased recognition of the complications, including excessive mucus formation, bladder rupture, calculi, dysplasia, and malignancy, metabolic acidosis, abnormalities of calcium metabolism,[1,7,12–17] and the hematuria–dysuria syndrome, metabolic alkalosis, and hypergastrinemia with the use of stomach, as discussed in Chapter 7.[18–20] The paradox of a concomitant nephroureterectomy and bladder augmentation with bowel became apparent as the complications of enterocystoplasty were more widely recognized. Concurrently, other techniques have been developed for the formation of a urothelial-lined neobladder, highlighting the appropriateness of other similar approaches. Autoaugmentation,[21–24] the most widely used urothelial-lined bladder augmentation, lacks a backing to the urothelium, whereas diverticulocystoplasty is limited to very few patients[25] and the use of urothelial-lined bowel and stomach segments are yet to be validated.[26–28] The ureter has all the appropriate layers and, not surprisingly, has become favored, particularly when there is high-grade vesicoureteric reflux;[1–3,5,7,15–17] in addition to improving the bladder, the procedure also eliminates the predisposition to urinary infection in the poorly draining ureter, without the need for ureteric reimplantation.

The first ureterocystoplasty was described by Eckstein and Martin, who reported a two-incision, extraperitoneal removal of a poorly functioning left kidney from a 7-month-old infant; they used a transverse bladder incision to incorporate the longitudinally incised ureter into the bladder. The authors, as confirmed by others, also showed that the procedure be can performed following a ureteric reimplantation:[16,29] the patient, now in his third decade, remains well (Etker, 1995, personal communication). Further experience with this procedure was not recorded until 1993. The operation was then described by Wolf and Turzan,[15] Bellinger,[17] Churchill *et al.*,[1] and Dewan *et al.* [2]. Generally, bladder capacity is increased by ureterocystoplasty, and continence and vesicoureteric reflux are improved. Unfortunately, the technique is only able to be used when the ureter is sufficiently dilated.[3,29] To produce enlarged ureters, attempts at dilation of a normal-sized ureter have been carried out experimentally, using a rabbit model, in which progressive ureteral dilation was achieved by means of saline injections through a subcutaneously implanted injection port; ureteric units were dilated by at least ten-fold, and augmentation cystoplasty performed with these dilated ureteral segments increased bladder capacity by an average of 260%.[30] Although this is interesting experimental work, it is not yet at the stage of clinical application.

Since Eckstein's paper, ureterocystoplasty has undergone many modifications. Originally, both the renal pelvis and the megaureter were thought necessary to ensure an adequate increase in bladder volume.[1,2,4–7,9,15,29,31,32] More recent studies have shown that the lower two-thirds of a dilated ureter provides a considerable increase in bladder capacity, allowing for preservation of the ipsilateral kidney.[6–8,17,29,32] This new development includes forming a transureteroureterostomy between the upper end of the ipsilateral ureter and the contralateral side. The lower two-thirds of the divided ureter is then used for the bladder augmentation; alternatively, the transected ureter is reimplanted into the bladder and the lower ureter is used for the augmentation if the ureter is long and tortuous. A further extension of this concept is the use of both ureters to enlarge the bladder,[6,31] or to facilitate ureterocystoplasty if the patient has only a single kidney.[33] Other less common applications of ureteric bladder augmentation have been in patients with massive reflux into nonfunctioning lower pole duplex systems in whom an obstructing ureterocele has resulted in bladder dysfunction.[6,32] Also, the upper ureter anastomosis to the contralateral side has been performed as a transureteropyeloplasty to relieve a pelviureteric junction obstruction on the side opposite to the ureterocystoplasty.[29]

Several authors have described the extraperitoneal approach recently highlighted by Wolf and Turzan.[15] The procedure uses the double incision suggested by Eckstein in 1973, which involves both lateral and Pfannenstiel incisions to mobilize the ureter of a non-functioning kidney and avoids the complications of the transperitoneal approach, minimizing postoperative pain and reducing the period of hospitalization.[1,2,5,15–17,32,34,35] Remaining in the extraperitoneal space also avoids the risk of contamination to existing ventriculoperitoneal shunts and facilitates subsequent peritoneal dialysis. Also, in girls, there is no pedicle to interfere with a Caesarean section if required in later years. The extraperitoneal approach can also be used to perform a combination of ureterocystoplasty and the transureteroureterostomy, by anastomosing the two ureters retroperitoneally.[34] Thus, the benefits of the extraperitoneal approach can be achieved while preserving the function of the ipsilateral kidney.

Of the large number of ureterocystoplasty cases thus far described, several have been 2 years of age or

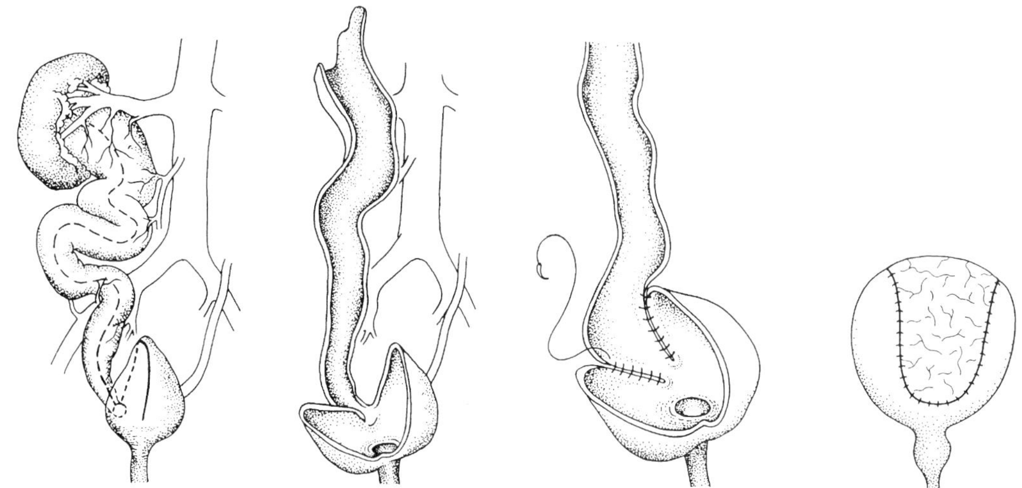

Figure 8.1 *A nonfunctioning kidney is removed, extraperitoneally, and the ureter configured and incorporated into the bladder. Reproduced with permission from Figure 1 in Dewan, P.A., Nicholls, E.A. and Goh, D.W. (1994) Ureterocystoplasty: an extraperitoneal, urothelial lined bladder augmentation technique.* European Urology, ***26***, *85–9.*

less, indicating the applicability to younger children,[1–3,5,7,16,17] whereas ileocystoplasty and gastrocystoplasty are rarely considered appropriate for the very young, although they have been used.[36,37]

PREOPERATIVE MANAGEMENT

It is important to ensure that the urethra is intubatable prior to performing a ureterocystoplasty, for two reasons: firstly, because intermittent catheterization should be anticipated after any bladder augmentation; and secondly because a suitable ureter will often be found in a boy who has previously had urethral obstruction. Nevertheless, many of these patients do not have a neurogenic sphincter, and therefore they will be able to void spontaneously after the procedure.

In anticipation of the unusual event of the ureter or its blood supply not being suitable, we prepare the patient for bladder augmentation with intestine.

Preoperative investigation includes assessment of the anatomy of the urinary tract, which should be fully reviewed prior to the procedure. This would include a cystogram (or ultrasound) and an intravenous urogram, antegrade pyelogram, or retrograde pyelogram, depending on requirements. It is also appropriate to assess the function of both kidneys with a nuclear medicine scan.

OPERATIVE TECHNIQUE

There are three main technique variations for the use of the ureter for bladder augmentation: extraperitoneal ureterocystoplasty is preferred when removing a nonfunctioning kidney; transperitoneal ureterocystoplasty with transureteroureterostomy when both kidneys should be preserved and other intraperitoneal procedures are required; or extraperitoneal ureterocystoplasty with transureteroureterostomy if both kidneys need to be preserved and intraperitoneal surgery is not necessary. The operative details are as follows.

Extraperitoneal ureterocystoplasty with nephrectomy (Fig. 8.1)[35]

With the child in a semilateral position, the kidney is mobilized through either a lateral, subcostal, muscle-cutting incision[2] or a dorsal lumbotomy.[5]

The ureteric blood supply is preserved during mobilization down to the pelvic brim, while preserving the peritoneum intact. The renal parenchyma is removed from the renal pelvis, the pelvis is oversewn and placed in the extraperitoneal space adjacent to the back of the bladder, and the nephrectomy wound is closed. The blood supply to the ureter and renal pelvis is dependent upon the perivesical vessels primarily, with additional branches from gonadal and lumbar periureteral tissues, therefore preservation of the gonadal vessels is one of the obvious goals. The mobilization of the ureter must keep an adequate 'ureteric mesentery,' as originally emphasized by Hendren in his papers describing megaureter reconstruction. The obliterated umbilical vessel on the affected side is divided to facilitate the preservation of the more medial vessels originating on the common and internal iliac vessels.

The bladder and mobilized ureter are then exposed via a transverse suprapubic skin incision and the ureter is further dissected extraperitoneally, taking care to preserve its lower lateral blood supply by avoiding dissection lateral to the ureteric orifice. When the ureter is sufficiently freed, the bladder is incised from the anterior bladder neck, over the dome, to the orifice of the nephrectomy ureter; the longitudinal incision of the ureter is facilitated by passage of a 12 FG catheter into the ureterocystoplasty ureter, and the ureter is opened along its anteromedial border. At the distal end of the ureter, the ureterovesical junction can either be left in continuity or incised longitudinally. If the original ureterovesical junction is left intact, the proximal ureter is opened distally to within 1 cm of the ureterovesical junction. Drainage of urine in the nondetubularized distal ureter is assured from both the 'ureteral' and the bladder lumens of the nonopened ureteral segment. If a previously reimplanted ureter is used, greater care should be taken not to disturb the lateral blood supply of the distal ureter.

Hinman has confirmed that reconfiguration of a bowel segment into a patch-like globular shape will increase the neobladder capacity after augmentation, and results in abolition of any inherent peristaltic activity. However, the ureter is often not of sufficient length to reconfigure and is only able to be sutured into the bladder as a clam cystoplasty. Therefore, the free edges of the inferiorly based ureteric flap are sutured to the edges of the incised bladder with a continuous 3/0 polyglycolic acid suture. As with all augmentation procedures, an intentional discrepancy between the perimeter of the native bladder and the reconfigured augmented ureteral segment is apparent at the time of the bladder closure. The ureteric tissue tolerates this discrepancy well, and the edges can be plicated to compensate for the difference.

The ureteral bladder augmentation can be combined with contralateral ureteric reimplantation, contralateral subureteral Teflon injection, contralateral ureteric stoma in transplanted patients, bladder neck continence procedure, or closure of the bladder neck. If the peritoneum is to be opened, as described in the following procedure, transureteroureterostomy, transureteropyelostomy and appendicovesicostomy can be performed.

Transperitoneal ureterocystoplasty with transureteroureterostomy (Fig. 8.2)

Access to the retroperitoneum, ureters, and kidneys is gained by mobilizing the mesentery of the small bowel and the right colon. The ureter to be used for the ureterocystoplasty is divided below the renal pelvis, at a distance which will facilitate the transureteroureterostomy. The upper end of the ureter is taken across to the contralateral upper ureter, after passing anterior to the aorta and inferior vena cava usually superior to the inferior mesenteric artery. The ureterocystoplasty is then performed with the lower end of the divided ureter in the manner described above. A Redivac drain is placed in both renal beds and a nephrostomy tube is inserted into the kidney from which the ureter has been taken for the ureterocystoplasty. Alternatively, a double J stent can be inserted during the ureteroureterostomy.

Extraperitoneal ureterocystoplasty with transureteroureterostomy[34]

The patient is placed in the lateral position and a standard nephrectomy-length skin crease incision is made below the twelfth rib; dissection is carried down

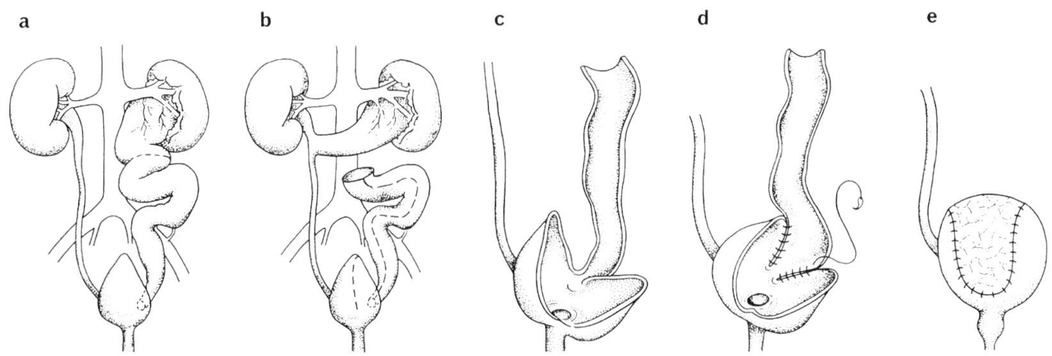

Figure 8.2 *Technique of ureteroplasty with transureteroureterostomy. (a) The dilated ureter is divided and allows for (b) anastomosis to the contralateral ureter. (c) The ectatic ureter is incised longitudinally, and (d, e) sutured into the bladder. Reproduced with permission from Figure 1 in Dewan, P.A.. (1996) Ureterocystoplasty with renal preservation in young infants.* Pediatric Surgery International, ***11****, 146.*[29]

through the muscle layers into the extraperitoneal plane and through Gerota's fascia. After inserting a Denis Browne ring-retractor, dissection is continued behind the peritoneum, anterior to the inferior vena cava and aorta, where the contralateral ureter is identified, and stay sutures are applied. A 1 cm, longitudinal incision is made in the far-side ureter and a length of the divided ureter is mobilized to facilitate a Y-shaped ureteroureterostomy. The end of the divided ureter is joined to the contralateral ureter on the far side; and the anastomosis is completed with a with a 5/0 polyglycolic acid suture. A double J stent can then be inserted or a ureteric catheter is placed from below during the bladder component of the operation. The lower ureter is then mobilized down to the pelvic brim, preserving its blood supply, and the lateral wound is closed after the insertion of a Redivac drain; the blood loss is usually minimal.

The patient is placed in the supine position and a modified Pfannenstiel incision is performed. The anterior wall of the bladder is mobilized, stay sutures are applied, and an incision is made from the anterior bladder neck to the urachus; dissection is then extended from the urachus to the orifice of the mobilized ureter, then longitudinally to the proximal end of the ureter. Two parallel suture lines are used to anastomose the right ureter to the opening in the bladder, thus completing the ureterocystoplasty. An 8 FG feeding tube is placed into the contralateral ureteric orifice and sutured with 4/0 chromic catgut. The bladder and abdominal wound are closed around a 10 FG Malecot catheter.

POSTOPERATIVE MANAGEMENT

A suprapubic catheter is placed in the bladder and removed when the patient is established on 3-hourly clean intermittent catheterization. Urine drainage postoperatively is achieved via a ureteric catheter which is removed after a cystogram 10 days postoperatively. A suprapubic tube can provide urine drainage in the postoperative period, either alone or in conjunction with a urethral catheter. We have employed a retroperitoneal drain following the procedure, and continued prophylactic antibiotics. In this period of wound healing and volume accommodation, the advantages of the choice of ureteric tissue became immediately apparent with the visible absence of mucus.

OUTCOME FOR URETEROCYSTOPLASTY

In 40 cases of ureterocystoplasty we have generally seen a satisfactory increasing bladder capacity while maintaining low bladder pressures (below 30 cmH_2O),[3] and achieving spontaneous voiding in many of the patients, most of whom remain infection free. Mucus formation has not been a problem and calculi have only been observed in one patient. Importantly, we do not anticipate that patients will have any increased susceptibility to malignancy. Follow-up of cases in the literature varies from 3 to 40 months, with no deterioration of renal function and an improvement in bladder volume and capacity, voiding ability, bladder stability, and continence usually recorded.[2–9,29,32,34]

Although ureterocystoplasty may not provide the same increase in bladder volume as can be expected from enterocystoplasty, intra-abdominal, bowel mucosal and nutritional consequences of routine cystoplasty are avoided. The procedure should be considered in the management of a high-pressure bladder with a refluxing megaureter.

REFERENCES

1. Churchill, B.M., Aliabadi, H., Landau, E.H. *et al.* (1993) Ureteral bladder augmentation. *Journal of Urology*, **150**, 716–20.
2. Dewan, P.A., Nicholls, E.A. and Goh, D.W. (1994) Ureterocystoplasty: an extraperitoneal, urothelial bladder augmentation technique. *European Urology*, **26**, 85–9.
3. Landau, E.H., Jayanthi, V.R., Khoury, A.E. *et al.* (1994) Bladder augmentation: ureterocystoplasty versus ileocystoplasty. *Journal of Urology*, **152**, 716–19.
4. Churchill, B.M., Jayathi, V.R., Landau, E.H. *et al.* (1995) Ureterocystoplasty: importance of the proximal blood supply. *Journal of Urology*, **154**, 197–8.
5. Reinberg, Y., Allen, R.C., Vaughn, M. *et al.* (1995) Nephrectomy combined with lower abdominal extraperitoneal ureteral bladder augmentation in the treatment of children with the vesicoureteral reflux dysplasia syndrome. *Journal of Urology,* **153,** 177–9.
6. Gosalbez, R. and Kim, C.O. (1996) Ureterocystoplasty with preservation of ipsilateral renal function. *Journal of Pediatric Surgery,* **31,** 970–5.
7. Hitchcock, R.J.I., Duffy, P.G. and Malone, P.S. (1994) Ureterocystoplasty: the 'bladder' augmentation of choice. *British Journal of Urology,* **73,** 575–9.
8. Ben-Chaim, J., Partin, A.W. and Jeffs, R.D. (1996) Ureteral bladder augmentation using the lower pole ureter of a duplicated system. *Urology,* **47,** 135–7.
9. Kim, C.O., Gosalbez, R. and Burke, G.W. (1997) Simultaneous ureterocystoplasty and living related renal transplantation. *Clinical Transplantation,* **10,** 333–6.
10. Hoover, D.L. and Duckett, J.W. (1982) Posterior urethral valves, unilateral reflux and renal dysplasia: a syndrome. *Journal of Urology,* **128,** 994–7.
11. Rittenberg, M.H., Hulbert, W.C., Snyder, H.M. *et al.* (1988) Protective factors in posterior urethral valves. *Journal of Urology,* **140,** 993–6.
12. Nurse, D.E. and Mundy, A.R. (1989) Metabolic complications of cystoplasty. *British Journal of Urology,* **63,** 165–70.
13. Mundy, A.R. and Nurse, D.E. (1992) Calcium balance, growth and skeletal mineralization in patients with cystoplasties. *British Journal of Urology,* **69,** 257–9.
14. Canning, D.A., Perman, J.A., Jeffs, R.D. *et al.* (1989) Nutritional consequences of bowel segments in the lower urinary tract. *Journal of Urology,* **142,** 509–11.
15. Wolf, J.S. and Turzan, C.W. (1993) Augmentation ureterocystoplasty. *Journal of Urology,* **149,** 1095–8.
16. Eckstein, H.B. and Martin, M.R.R. (1973) Uretero-cystoplastik. *Actuelle Urologie,* **4,** 255–7.
17. Bellinger, M.F. (1993) Ureterocystoplasty: a unique method for vesical augmentation in children. *Journal of Urology,* **149,** 811–13.
18. Gosalbez, R., Woodard, J.R., Broecker, B.H. *et al.* (1993) Metabolic complications of the use of stomach for urinary reconstruction. *Journal of Urology,* **150,** 710–12.
19. Nguyen, D.H., Bain, M.A., Salmonson, K.L. *et al.* (1993) The syndrome of dysuria and hematuria in pediatric urinary reconstruction with stomach. *Journal of Urology,* **150,** 707–9.
20. Kinahan, T.J., Khoury, A.E., McLorie, G.A. *et al.* (1992) Omeprazole in post-gastrocystoplasty metabolic alkalosis and aciduria. *Journal of Urology,* **147,** 435–7.

21. Cartwright, P.C. and Snow, B.W. (1989) Bladder autoaugmentation: early clinical experience. *Journal of Urology,* **142,** 505–8.
22. Cartwright, P.C. and Snow, B.W. (1989) Bladder autoaugmentation: partial detrusor excision to augment the bladder without use of bowel. *Journal of Urology,* **142,** 1050–3.
23. Kennelly, M.J., Gormley, E.A. and McGuire, E.J. (1994) Early clinical experience with adult bladder auto-augmentation. *Journal of Urology,* **152,** 303–6.
24. Ehrlich, R.M. and Gershman, A. (1993) Laparoscopic seromyotomy (auto-augmentation) for non-neurogenic neurogenic bladder in a child: initial case report. *Urology,* **42,** 175–8.
25. Dewan, P.A. and Lorenz, C. (1994) Bladder incorporation of large paraureteric diverticula: diverticulocystoplasty. *Australian and New Zealand Journal of Surgery,* **64,** 731–4.
26. Dewan, P.A. and Stefanek, W. (1994) Autoaugmentation colocystoplasty: a case report. *Pediatric Surgery International,* **9,** 526–8.
27. Gonzalez, R., Buson, H., Reid, C. *et al.* (1995) Seromuscular colocystoplasty lined with urothelium: experience with 16 patients. *Urology,* **45,** 124–9.
28. Dewan, P.A. and Stefanek, W. (1994) Autoaugmentation gastrocystoplasty: early clinical results. *British Journal of Urology,* **74,** 460–4.
29. Dewan, P.A. (1996) Ureterocystoplasty with renal preservation in young infants. *Pediatric Surgery International,* **11,** 146–9.
30. Cilento, B.G., Lailas, N.G., Retik, A.B. *et al.* (1995) Progressive dilatation for subsequent uretero-cystoplasty. *Journal of Urology,* **153** (Suppl.), 57.
31. Ahmed, S., Neel, K.F. and Sen, S. (1998) Tandem ureterocystoplasty. *Australian and New Zealand Journal of Surgery,* **68,** 203–5.
32. Zubieta, R., deBadiola, F., Escala, J.M. *et al.* (1998) Clinic and urodynamic evaluation after uretero-cystoplasty with different amounts of tissue. *Pediatrics,* **102** (3(2)), 848.
33. Dewan, P.A. and Condron, S.K. (1999) Ureterocystoplasty with a single kidney. *Pediatric Surgery International,* **15**, 413–14.
34. Dewan, P.A. and Condron, S.K. (1999) Extraperitoneal ureterocystoplasty with transureteroureterostomy. *Urology,* **53** (3), 634–6.
35. Dewan, P.A., Nicholls, E.A. and Goh, D.W. (1994) Ureterocystoplasty: an extraperitoneal, urothelial lined bladder augmentation technique. *European Urology,* **26,** 85–9.
36. Dykes, E.H. and Ransley, P.G. (1992) Gastrocystoplasty in children. *British Journal of Urology,* **69,** 91–5.
37. Krishna, A. and Gough, D.C.S. (1994) Evaluation of augmentation cystoplasty in childhood with reference to vesicoureteric reflux and urinary infection. *British Journal of Urology,* **74,** 465–8.

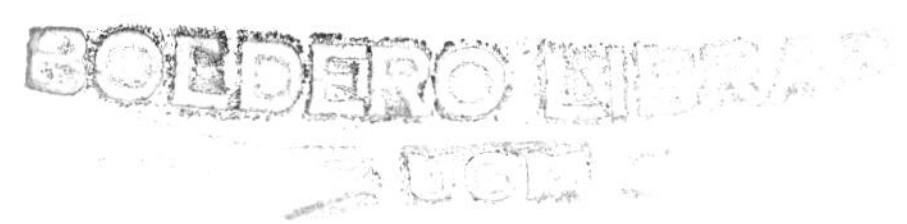

9

Seromuscular enterocystoplasty

JOAO LUIZ PIPPI SALLE AND ROMAN JEDNAK

INTRODUCTION

Another alternative to bladder augmentation is the use of demucosalized intestine or stomach. The intestinal or gastric mucosa is removed and the seromuscular layer is used for bladder or ureteral substitution. This so-called seromuscular enterocystoplasty or gastrocystoplasty was initially used in animal experimentation.

The first description of seromuscular enterocystoplasty was published in 1955.[1,2] Seromuscular segments of ileum and colon were used for bladder augmentation in dogs undergoing subtotal cystectomy. The animals were augmented with reversed pedicle grafts of seromuscular segments of ileum or colon (serosal side facing the bladder lumen) or with identical nonreversed segments stripped of either mucosa or of both mucosa and submucosa (demucosalized area facing the bladder lumen). The groups of animals undergoing reversed ileal or colonic seromuscular enterocystoplasty had postoperative cystograms showing 'normal-functioning bladders.' Bladder capacity was above preoperative values and the entire segment used for augmentation was covered by urothelium in 7 to 10 days following surgery. In the original description, these segments were covered by epithelium that was 'indistinguishable from normal bladder epithelium.' In addition, the segments were characterized by 'the plexiform arrangement of muscle bundles indistinguishable from the plexiform arrangement of the detrusor muscle of the normal canine bladder.' The animals also failed to absorb urine electrolytes and had very little mucus or bacteria in their urine. In the group of animals in which only the mucosa was removed, leaving the submucosa facing the bladder lumen, the intestinal mucosa was found to regenerate in every instance. Furthermore, several weeks later, the bladders in these animals were found to be identical to those of the control group that had undergone standard ileocystoplasty or colocystoplasty. The group of animals in which both the mucosa and submucosa were removed did not regenerate intestinal mucosa, and although the augmented area was covered with urothelium, biopsies showed areas of 'osteoid formation and intraluminal adhesions;' contraction of the seromuscular segment was not mentioned. The authors concluded that reversed demucosalized bowel was the best material for augmentation. The importance of this contribution was clearly recognized by the urologic community and, in 1955, this work was awarded first prize in the essay competition sponsored annually by The American Urological Association. The authors later reported the use of reversed demucosalized augmentation cystoplasty in four patients with reduced bladder capacity secondary to partial cystectomy, myelomeningocele, idiopathic contracted bladder, and interstitial cystitis. The augmented segment contracted completely in one patient, and two patients with myelomeningocele were reportedly continent, despite bladder capacities of only 130–150 cm^3. Data were not available on the remaining patient and no long-term follow-up was reported.[3]

Martin, in 1959, reported on the use of ileal seromuscular segments which were harvested with small urothelial-free grafts in dogs undergoing partial cystectomy and nonreversed demucosalized ileocystoplasty. The urothelial-free grafts were placed on one group of bowel segments. Three weeks postoperatively, the augmented/grafted animals were reported to have normal cystograms and cystometrograms, with normal urothelium covering the augmented segments.[4]

Campbell, in 1957, reported the case of a 57-year-old man who had undergone reversed demucosalized bowel augmentation of his bladder. Postoperatively, apart from recording that the patient developed a draining sinus, no data describing the functional result were reported.[5]

The need for total removal of the muscularis mucosa along with the mucosa to avoid enteric mucosal regeneration was emphasized by Torbey and Mozden.[6] The authors utilised seromuscular segments of ileum for the construction of a Bricker ileal conduit. Regeneration of the intestinal mucosa occurred when the muscularis mucosa was not removed, but did not occur when both the mucosa and submucosa were removed. The investigators also studied a group of animals in which half of the segment had both mucosa and submucosa removed, and half was left intact. Interestingly, if not splinted, a tendency to constriction was observed in the portion of the segment from which both the mucosa and submucosa had been removed.

Other investigators have attempted to avoid the use of intestinal mucosa in bladder augmentation. Koontz *et al.*, in 1970, reported on experimental work in dogs that underwent subtotal cystectomy and had the vesical remnant covered with the serosal surface of the intact sigmoid. These authors observed 'migration of transitional cell epithelium across the serosal surface of the sigmoid colon by the fourth to seventh postoperative day.' By day 30, 'the entire serosal surface was covered with this epithelium.' Significant complications were observed in these animals, including vesicocolonic fistulas, calculus formation, and osseous formation predominantly at the junction of the bladder and bowel serosa.[7] Cheng *et al.* performed the same experiment in two dogs and obtained similar results.[8] Little interest in seromuscular enterocystoplasty was evident until the late 1980s, when Oesch (1988) and Salle *et al.* (1990) revisited this form of bladder augmentation.[9,10] In Oesch's experimental work, seromuscular enterocystoplasty was performed in seven rats by excising the mucosa of a cecal segment and suturing it to the bladder following subtotal cystectomy. The author reported very good results, as complete urothelial epithelialization without patch contraction was observed. Salle *et al.*, in 1990, reported different results in dogs undergoing ileal or sigmoid colon seromuscular enterocystoplasty.[11] The ileum or sigmoid colon was stripped of both mucosa and submucosa and the seromuscular segment was used for a clam type of bladder augmentation (Plate 1). Postoperatively, bladder decompression was maintained by cystostomy drainage for a period of 8 to 10 days, and the animals were sacrificed 8 weeks later. The animals voided normally and the urine was clear in the postoperative period. No stones developed and normal amounts of mucus were present, but the patch was severely contracted in all animals (Plate 2). Histological examination revealed complete urothelial coverage of the seromuscular segment with severe contraction and significant fibrosis (Plate 3). The authors' hypotheses for the etiology of the contraction were: (a) fibrosis was chemically induced by the chronic contact of the rough seromuscular layer with urine; (b) ischemia ocurred during the removal of the mucosa and submucosa; (c) chronic urinary infection led to inflammation and scarring of the seromuscular patch; (d) there was prolonged postoperative bladder decompression. During the presentation of their paper, the authors reported preliminary results using autoaugmentation in association with seromuscular enterocystoplasty.[10] The idea was to prevent urine contact with the seromuscular segment, and possibly avoid its contraction by maintaining an intact bladder epithelium. This technique of autoaugmentation enterocystoplasty, using both colon and stomach, is further discussed in Chapters 11–13. Subsequent examination revealed that the interposed segment underwent fibrosis and shrinkage.[11]

FIBROSIS OF THE SEROMUSCULAR SEGMENT

Motley *et al.*, in 1990, performed seromuscular sigmoid cystoplasty in calves. The sigmoid mucosa was removed leaving the muscularis layer exposed and the segment was then used for a cup-shaped cystoplasty. Urothelial epithelialization occurred in all animals but, as previously reported, all augmented bladders experienced significant contraction and fibrosis. Particular attention was given to vascular histology and no evidence of vascular thrombosis was observed. The authors also noted progressive collagen deposition in the augmented segment. Regeneration of colonic mucosa (nests of mucosa) took place in all cases.[12]

In 1991, reversed seromuscular enterocystoplasty was performed in rats by de Badiola *et al.*[13] Both the mucosa and submucosa of the sigmoid colon were mechanically removed and the serosa and muscularis layers were used for a reversed augmenting cystoplasty. A complication rate of 42% was encountered and included mainly bladder stones (25%) and colovesical fistulas (12%). The remaining rats had a significant increase in bladder capacity, with transitional epithelialization of the serosal layer as early as 5 days postoperatively. No regrowth of enteric mucosa was noted. There was no evidence of an inflammatory infiltrate or fibrosis of the sigmoid muscularis. In areas where the intestinal mucosa had been completely denuded, the muscular wall was covered by a layer of granulation tissue that contained hemosiderin-laden macrophages and foreign-body reaction; this layer was covered by regenerating mesothelium or by adherent peritoneum. Patch size was also measured at the time of operation and at the time of sacrifice (mean time 30 days) in 26 rats, and an increase in the surface area from 1.82 cm^2 to 2.3 cm^2 was noted. The absence of contraction of the seromuscular patch could be explained by the placement of the serosal side of the segment such that it faced the bladder lumen, thereby preventing the contact of urine with the rough muscular layer. Similarly, Oesch did not observe severe fibrosis of the seromuscular segment, and speculated that contraction was less likely to occur in small animals.[9] Cheng *et al.* performed reversed seromuscular ileocystoplasty in dogs and observed significant patch contraction.[8] Urine cultures were negative in all animals. They concluded that fibrosis of the seromuscular patch was probably multifactorial, and that the trauma of mucosal stripping seems to have major importance in this phenomenon. They agreed with previous researchers who speculated that their differing results could be due to the different sizes of the experimental animals.

Long *et al.* in 1992, further studied this question and devised a model of seromuscular colocystoplasty in dogs, which included the performance of a proximal urinary diversion (bilateral ureterostomies).[14] Both mucosal and submucosal layers were removed in eight of nine dogs. Animals were observed for 1, 2 and 4 weeks postoperatively, and then sacrificed. Diminished bladder capacity was observed in all animals (from 409 cm^3 preoperatively to 80 cm^3 postoperatively), but all patches remained viable and well vascularized. The authors concluded that the presence of urine in the bladder after seromuscular enterocystoplasty was unlikely to be the sole cause of patch contraction.

Removal of the muscularis mucosa and submucosa during preparation of the intestinal seromuscular segment seems to lead to contraction of the patch. Buson *et al.* in 1994, compared results using seromuscular sigmoid segments with and without submucosa in dogs.[15] They reported a decreased bladder capacity in animals augmented with seromuscular segments deprived of submucosa. Histological examination of these specimens revealed contraction of the patch and subepithelial fibrosis of the lamina propria. Dogs in which the submucosa was maintained had a significant increase in bladder capacity with minimal fibrosis of the patch. Other investigators have also reported minimal shrinkage of the patch when only the mucosal layer is removed. Regrowth of intestinal mucosa has often been observed in these situations, however, and is of concern.[16,17]

Prolonged bladder decompression following seromuscular enterocystoplasty may play an important etiologic role in augmenting segment contraction.[8,10,] In Gonzalez's clinical experience, this issue receives important consideration. Postoperatively, patients are kept with a permanently distended bladder, allowing close contact of the intact urothelium with the seromuscular segment. Patch collapse is thereby prevented. For this reason, Gonzalez avoids performing additional procedures that require entering the bladder lumen, as this may lead to urinary leakage and difficulty in keeping the bladder distended.[18]

We recently developed an experimental model in rabbits to evaluate the effects of urine contact with seromuscular segments.[19] A segment of gastric fundus, based on the right gastroepiploic artery, was manually demucosalized. The raw surface of the gastric seromuscular segment was then sutured to the anterior abdominal wall. The animals were observed and explored 3 weeks postoperatively. The seromuscular patch was measured, carefully separated from the peritoneum, and biopsies were taken from the borders. The patch dimensions remained unchanged and no evidence of fibrosis was seen on histological examination. The patch was then used for bladder augmentation without postoperative urinary drainage. After 4 weeks of exposure to urine, all the gastric flaps were contracted and histologically fibrotic.

From this study, we concluded that vascular compromise did not appear to play a primary role in the fate of the flaps. Direct contact with urine was probably responsible for the fibrosis and contraction of pedicled de-epithelialized gastric flaps following bladder augmentation.[19] This conclusion, however, cannot be extended to de-epithelialized intestinal segments, which may suffer from compromized vascular supply following removal of the submucosa. Nevertheless, the study clearly demonstrates the deleterious effects of urine contact with the raw muscular layer.

CONCLUSIONS

Seromuscular enterocystoplasty may be a significant technical advancement in the treatment of patients requiring bladder augmentation, as normal urothelial coverage is achieved. Contraction and regrowth of intestinal mucosa in the augmenting seromuscular segment, however, remain significant complications. The use of this technique in combination with autoaugmentation avoids direct contact with urine, which may be an important etiological factor for patch contraction. In addition, preservation of the submucosa appears to play an important role in maintaining elasticity and preventing shrinkage of the seromuscular segment, but may promote the undesirable complication of intestinal mucosal regrowth. Careful removal of remaining mucosal islands and treatment with urea and protamine sulfate have diminished, but not avoided, enteric mucosal regrowth. Although these techniques have now been used clinically, long-term follow-up is still not available. Further studies are necessary if we are to understand how to overcome related complications and recommend this technique routinely for bladder augmentation.

REFERENCES

1. Shoemaker, W.C. (1955) Reversed seromuscular grafts in urinary tract reconstruction. *Journal of Urology*, **74**, 453–75.
2. Shoemaker, W.C. and Marucci, H. (1955) The experimental use of seromuscular grafts in bladder reconstruction. *Journal of Urology*, **73**, 314–21.
3. Shoemaker, W.C., Bower, R. and Long, D. Jr (1957) A new technique for bladder reconstruction. *Surgery, Gynecology and Obstetrics*, **105**, 645–9.
4. Martin, L. (1959) Urothelial lined segment as a bladder replacement: experimental observations and brief review of literature. *Journal of Urology*, **82**, 633–50.
5. Campbell, E.W. (1957) Reconstruction of the bladder with a seromuscular graft. *Journal of Urology*, **78**, 236–41.

6. Torbey, P.K. and Mozden, P.J. (1966) Experimental use of a seromuscular segment of ileum as a urinary bladder substitution: technique, histologic change and absorptive capacity. *Annals of Surgery,* **163**, 589–96.
7. Koontz, W.W., Prout, G.R. and Mackler, M.A. (1970) Bladder regeneration following serosal colocystoplasty. *Investigative Urology,* **8,** 170–6.
8. Cheng, E., Rento, R., Grayhack, J.T. *et al.* (1994) Reversed seromuscular flaps in the urinary tract in dogs. *Journal of Urology,* **152**, 2252–7.
9. Oesch, I. (1988) Neurothelium in bladder augmentation. An experimental study in rats. *European Urology,* **14**, 328–9.
10. Salle, J.L., Fraga, J.C., Lucin, A.A. *et al.* (1990) Seromuscular enterocystoplasty in dogs. *Journal of Urology,* **144**, 454–6.
11. Salle, J.L., Ganesan, G. and Rink, R.C. (1989) Autoaugmentation colocystoplasty in dogs (unpublished data).
12. Motley, R.C., Montgomery, B.T., Zollman, P.E. *et al.* (1990) Augmentation cystoplasty utilizing de-epithelialized sigmoid colon: a preliminary study. *Journal of Urology,* **143**, 1257–60.
13. de Badiola, F., Manivel, J.C. and Gonzalez, R. (1992) Seromuscular enterocystoplasty in rats. *Journal of Urology,* **146,** 559–62.
14. Long, R.J., Buson, H., Manivel, J.C. *et al.* (1992) Seromuscular enteroplasty in dogs. *Journal of Urology,***147**, 430A.
15. Buson, H., Manivel, J.C., Dayane, M. *et al.* (1994) Seromuscular colocystoplasty lined with urothelium: experimental study. *Urology,* **44,** 743–8.
16. Lutz, N. and Frey, P. (1995) Enterocystoplasty using modified pedicled, tubularised, de-epithelialised sigmoid patches in the mini-pig model. *Journal of Urology,* **154,** 893–8.
17. Dewan, P.A., Close, C.E., Ashwood, P.J. *et al.* (1996) Enteric mucosal regrowth after bladder augmentation using demucosalised gut segments. *Journal of Urology*, **158**, 1141–6.
18. Gonzalez, R., Buson, H., Churphena, R. and Reiberg, Y. (1995) Seromuscular colocystoplasty lined with urothelium: experience with 16 patients. *Urology*, **45**,124–9.
19. Salle, J.L., Homayoon, K., Agarwal, S.K. *et al.* (1997) Determining factor in the contraction of de-epithelialised gastric flap for bladder augmentation. *Journal of Urology,* **157,** 769A.

10

Autoaugmentation cystoplasty

PATRICK CARTWRIGHT AND BRENT SNOW

INTRODUCTION

Many anomalies and disorders of childhood may result in significant reduction of bladder compliance with resultant incontinence, hydronephrosis, infection, and progressive renal insufficiency. Following management with anticholinergics or smooth muscle relaxants, along with modifications in voiding pattern or intermittent catheterization, the preferred management for a significant problem with bladder compliance becomes surgical. The goals of surgical intervention to augment the bladder include: (a) providing adequate storage capacity; (b) achieving low filling pressures; (c) ensuring spontaneous emptying; and (d) incurring minimal morbidity. While enterocystoplasty has been widely applied as a bladder augmentation procedure, the significant associated morbidities, as have been discussed in previous chapters, prompted many surgeons to seek alternatives for bladder augmentation.[1–3]

Attempts at various alternative methods of augmentation can be cited. Both natural and synthetic materials have been used experimentally to enlarge the bladder.[4–8] However, the naturally occurring bladder diverticulum seen in patients with chronic bladder outlet obstruction increases low-pressure bladder storage, which leads us to postulate that a surgically created, large-mouthed diverticulum might fill the requirements for successful bladder augmentation.[9,10]

The concept of removing bladder muscle from the dome of the bladder while leaving epithelium intact was thus developed and termed 'autoaugmentation,' because no extravesical tissue is utilized in the technique (Plate 4). Since the first inception of the operation, various names have been applied to this procedure, including partial detrusorectomy, autocystoplasty, detrusor myomectomy, and vesicomyomectomy. There has now been a modicum of experience reported using the technique of bladder autoaugmentation in the setting of poor bladder compliance.

ANIMAL MODELS

We initially evaluated the concept of autoaugmentation in a canine model with normal bladder function.[9] Cystometric evaluation and cystography were performed before and after the operative procedure. Detrusor was removed from the upper half of the

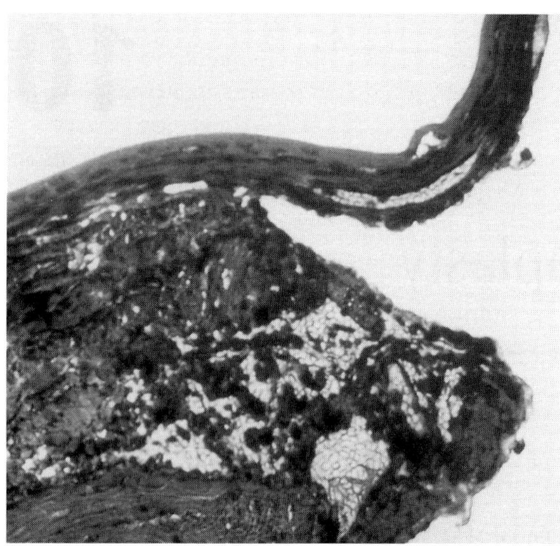

Figure 10.1 *Bladder wall following autoaugmentation in a rabbit. At the top are the remaining urothelium and lamina propria, and below is the intact bladder wall. (Reprinted from H. Johnson, M.D., Courtesy of* Urology*).*

bladder; the dissection proved to be simple, with the underlying urothelium remaining intact (Fig. 10.1). Small vessels could be identified within the remaining epithelial bulge, through which flow was revealed, using fluorescein perfusion. The bladder was drained with an indwelling catheter for 7 days, and the animals were evaluated when sacrificed at 2, 4 and 6 weeks following surgery.

The bladder appeared intact at sacrifice, without perforation or necrosis. Cystograms confirmed a diffuse bulge at the dome of the bladder, while histologically, bladder epithelium and lamina propria were intact, with a hypercellular layer of collagen and fibroblasts present just outside this bladder epithelium. Urodynamic evaluation postoperatively showed variable changes from the preoperative status, with little change in capacity, but generally improved compliance. Such variable urodynamic changes were anticipated, in that these dogs did not have neurogenic bladders, but normal, highly compliant bladders preoperatively. The technique proved to be technically feasible.

In another animal model, Johnson *et al.* performed the autoaugmentation procedure in 32 rabbits, removing the detrusor cuff in half the animals and leaving it intact in the remainder.[11] They consistently created a large diverticulum with a 17.2% net increase in surface area of the bladder epithelium, which was reproduced in a reduced functional capacity model, wherein one-third of the bladder was resected before autoaugmentation was undertaken.

Finally, in a sheep model (without neurogenic bladder), Dewan and associates performed autoaugmentation and covered the epithelial segment with omentum.[12] This resulted in no long-term augmenting effect, but again the starting-point was that of a normally compliant bladder, not one with reduced compliance.

TECHNIQUE

The technique of autoaugmentation has now been applied reasonably broadly to the care of patients.[13] The preparation, operative technique, and postoperative management are all generally straightforward.[14]

A mechanical and antibiotic bowel preparation is undertaken in all patients preoperatively, anticipating possible enterocystoplasty. A urine sample is obtained via catheter and cultured. After reviewing the procedure with the patient and parents, it is put to the parents that, if autoaugmentation is chosen, this will be attempted in the first instance, but that if the intraoperative result appears unsatisfactory, enterocystoplasty will subsequently be performed.

The patient is positioned supine and draped, with access to the urethra. A double lumen urodynamic catheter is placed via the urethra, and secured to the thigh to prevent its dislodgement. We originally placed a Foley catheter for filling and emptying of the bladder during dissection; however, it now seems best to perform intraoperative cystometric evaluation to assess changes resulting from the dissection.

After a low midline skin incision, the fascia is divided and extraperitoneal exposure of the bladder is obtained. Sterile tubing is run off the field from the double lumen catheter to the urodynamics equipment, and a pressure/volume bladder filling curve is generated before the detrusor is split. This initial tracing is then compared to those obtained after the dissection to see whether the filling curve indicates a significant improvement in compliance.

A circular, fixed retractor is preferred for this procedure. Following exposure of the bladder, an Allis clamp is used to grasp the anterior bladder wall near the dome and rotate it inferiorly. The peritoneal reflection on the posterior bladder wall is thus exposed, and can be dissected off the bladder to create an adequate field for autoaugmentation.

With the bladder dome now fully exposed, a longitudinal detrusor incision is made over the dome from anterior to posterior. The initial incision is made with electrocautery and carried through three-quarters of the bladder wall thickness. As the uroepithelial layer is approached, it is safer to use a hemostat to dissect under the final muscle bundles and expose the actual epithelium. Keeping the epithelium intact greatly facilitates dissection. As the last detrusor bundles are cauterized, the epithelium begins to bulge (Plate 5). The idea is to make enough of an incision that, with lateral mobilization, detrusor can be removed from over the superior half of the bladder, thus generating an augmenting bulge of urothelium.

Once the epithelium is exposed through the midline detrusor incision, Allis clamps are used to grasp detrusor edges, and the dissection is extended laterally in both directions. Bladder filling and emptying are crucial to maximize the ease of dissection, and are done through the urodynamic catheter. With optimal distension of the underlying epithelium and counteraction using Allis clamps, as mentioned, the dissection can be carried out with either a fine-tipped tenotomy scissor to gently spread and snip muscle bands, or with a fine right-angled hemostat. Detrusor fibers are separated from the underlying bladder epithelium in this fashion (Plate 6). Unless there is severe trabeculation and scarring from previous surgery, this is a technically feasible but tedious procedure. Care should be taken not to overspread between epithelium and bladder muscle, or to inadvertently lift the fibres too abruptly away from epithelium, as this will result in tears. Optimal magnification is very helpful.

If the dissection becomes particularly difficult in one area, it is wise to move to a different spot and work back toward this more adherent area, thus gaining a different angle on the dissection. As the autoaugmentation progresses, the Allis clamps must be advanced laterally in order to keep efficient countertraction applied. There will be small vessels perforating from detrusor into the lamina propria, and these will need cautery for maintenance of hemostasis. Some areas of the bladder favor easy dissection when the bladder is relatively tense, while in others the bladder must be partially emptied for the dissection to be optimally carried out. The bladder can be filled and emptied through the urodynamic tubing, as needed, to maintain appropriate bladder fullness.

With dissection at the dome, caution is needed to avoid the urachus. It is best ligated, with dissection carried out around its base. If a small perforation occurs there, or in any area, it may be oversewn with a 5/0 or 6/0 absorbable suture. If the perforation occurs at the very edge of dissection, if necessary a small amount of muscle is left in place around the site of perforation and the dissection is continued beyond this. This rim of muscle is helpful in securing sutures when closing these small perforations. Despite careful dissection, perforations can occur, and do not seem to prejudice the outcome or significantly change the postoperative course if ligated and dealt with intraoperatively. Once the dissection seems to encompass around one-half of the bladder surface, the bulging epithelium should distend well beyond its original confines (Plate 7). At this point, a new pressure/volume filling curve is generated, and compared to the predissection curve. If bladder volume at pressures of 20 cmH_2O and 40 cmH_2O is not significantly improved following this dissection, further dissection is contemplated. Although there are no precise guidelines for success, we look for at least a 30–50% increase in volumes at these various filling pressures. If little change in compliance and capacity is noted, the urothelium is removed and an enterocystoplasty is performed. Since the bladder has already been opened widely during the dissection, no difficulty is encountered in accomplishing an enterocystoplasty.

On the other hand, if capacity and compliance changes are encouraging, either bilateral or unilateral psoas hitches may be performed to straighten the posterior wall of the bladder and prevent adherence of the raw edges of dissected detrusor to the abdominal wall or other adjacent structures. Such adherence could limit expansion of the new autoaugmented segment of the bladder.

The dissected detrusor muscle is excised with electrocautery to prevent re-adherence to the urothelial bulge. The bladder is drained using either a urethral catheter or via a suprapubic tube placed through the intact lower portion of the bladder. Alternatively, Landa and Moorhead described leaving a small detrusor cap superiorly in the middle of the dissection and bringing the suprapubic tube through this area.[14] A Penrose drain is placed in the perivesical space, and the incision is closed in a standard fashion.

There are patients in whom autoaugmentation is technically difficult. Heavily trabeculated bladders are challenging because of the irregularity associated with multiple diverticula. When dissecting under trabecular fibers between diverticula, perforation occurs if the hemostat is overadvanced. Autoaugmentation is also technically more problematic in patients born with bladder exstrophy or following multiple operations. We opt for enterocystoplasty when technical factors preclude autoaugmentation.

It is possible to perform ureteral reimplantation for reflux or obstruction simultaneously with autoaugmentation. This has been accomplished in two different ways. An extravesical reimplant can be performed initially and followed by autoaugmentation. Alternatively, the bladder may be opened in a low transverse fashion anteriorly, intravesical reimplants being performed through this incision. The incision may then be closed and the autoaugmentation carried out in the usual fashion over the dome. We have also performed a simultaneous Mitrofanoff procedure to create a catheterizable abdominal stoma using the appendix. Other simultaneous procedures reported have included periurethral collagen injection, closure of vesicostomy, artificial urinary sphincter, and urethral sling procedures.

Some points of postoperative management should be made. Patients with intraoperative mucosal leaks may have extravasation for as long as 3.5 weeks. A Penrose drain is left in place until this extravasation ceases. The suprapubic Foley catheter generally drains until a cystogram has confirmed no leakage 7 to 10 days following surgery. Four patients showed new reflux after autoaugmentation. Resolution has now occurred in all but one. Once the catheter is removed, intermittent catheterization is reinstituted. Beginning 24 hours postoperatively, we have either caused persistent slight intravesical pressure elevation by leaving the catheter drainage tube 20 cm above bladder height (over the bedside rail), or we have intermittently irrigated the catheter with a fixed amount of saline and temporarily (for 30 minutes) clamped the tube. This induces modest distension and avoids contracted healing. We have seen no bladder rupture or perforation. Patients remain on antibiotic prophylaxis for at least 3 months postoperatively, as they seem to be vulnerable to infections over this period of time.

CLINICAL EXPERIENCE

In our experience, the clinical outcome of patients undergoing bladder autoaugmentation has been mixed. In some, the results are quite encouraging, while in others they are not.[13] Thirty patients are now available for review, with follow-up of greater than 1 year.

All patients had a history of poorly compliant bladders preoperatively, and had failed nonoperative management, including intermittent catheterization and various medications directed at improving bladder compliance. The primary diseases included myelomeningocele (19), tethered cord (2), posterior urethral obstruction (2), sacral agenesis (2), Hinman syndrome (2), and undetermined neuropathic bladder (3). Patients demonstrated the usual range of clinical problems associated with diminished bladder compliance and hyperreflexia, including incontinence (28), recurrent urinary tract infections (21), hydroureteronephrosis (19), vesicoureteral reflux (12), and renal insufficiency (10).

Our approach to patient selection has changed during the past several years. Earlier in the series, we considered performing the procedure in any patient needing enterocystoplasty; this included our first ten patients.[13] Following this initial experience, it seemed that the most appropriate patients, in terms of likelihood of success, might be those with distinctly poor compliance but initial preoperative bladder capacity of around 75% or greater for their expected capacity at that age. Those with more severe reduction in bladder capacity were considered instead for initial enterocystoplasty. Over the past 5 years as many patients have undergone initial enterocystoplasty or gastrocystoplasty as have been treated primarily with autoaugmentation.

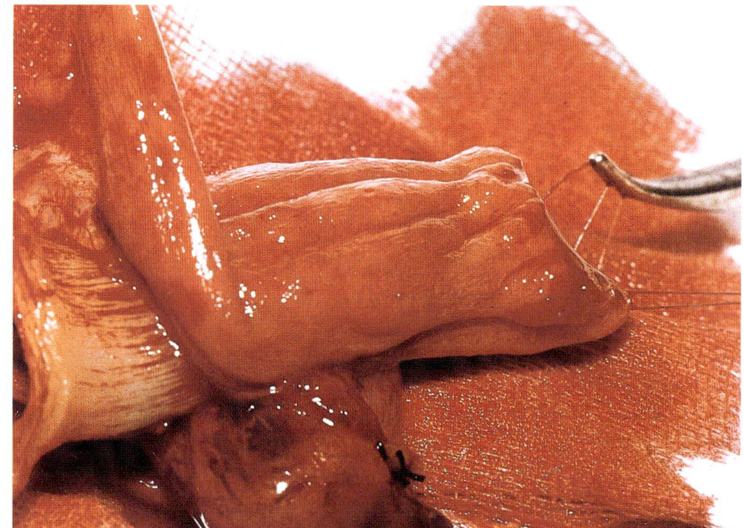

(a)

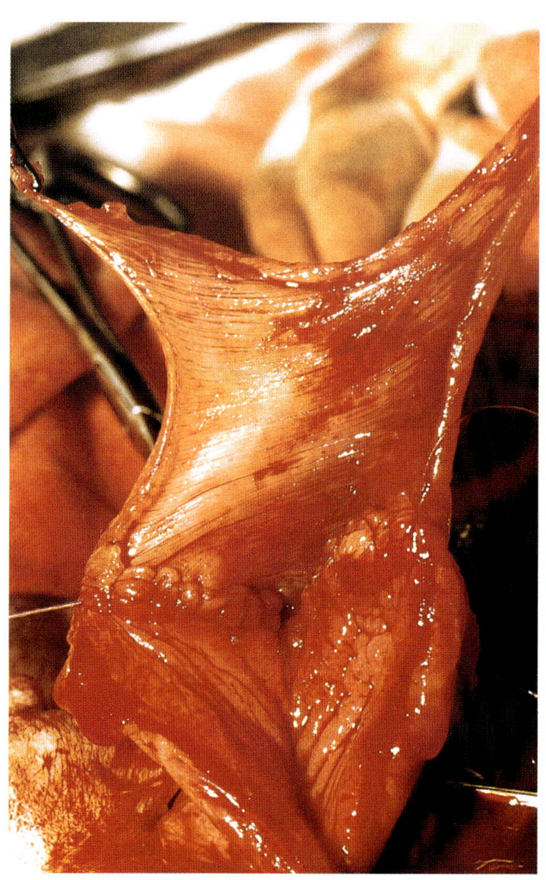

(b)

Plate 1 *(a) Mucosa and submucosa being stripped from the sigmoid seromuscular layer. (b) Bladder being augmented with sigmoid seromuscular segment.*

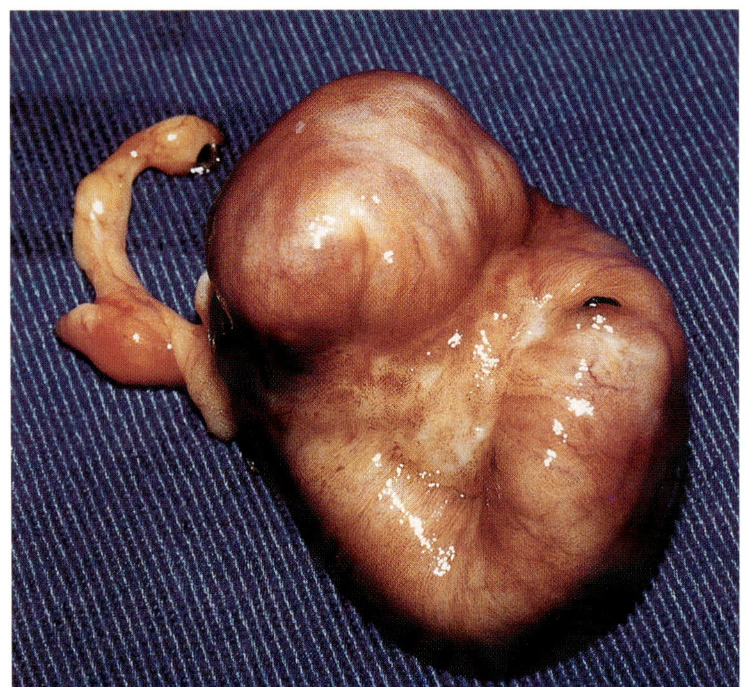

Plate 2 *Severe contraction of the seromuscular patch used in augmentation which is about one-fifth of its original size.*

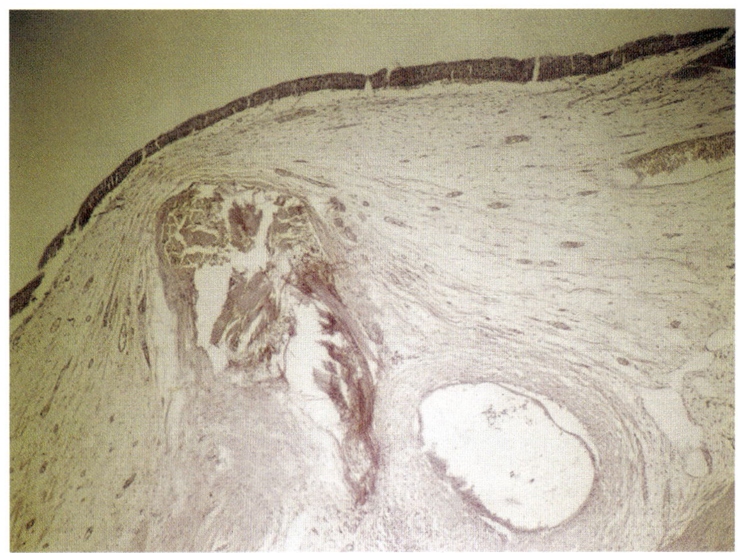

Plate 3 *Histological section of the augmented bladder. The seromuscular segment shows severe fibrosis and is covered with transitional epithelium.*

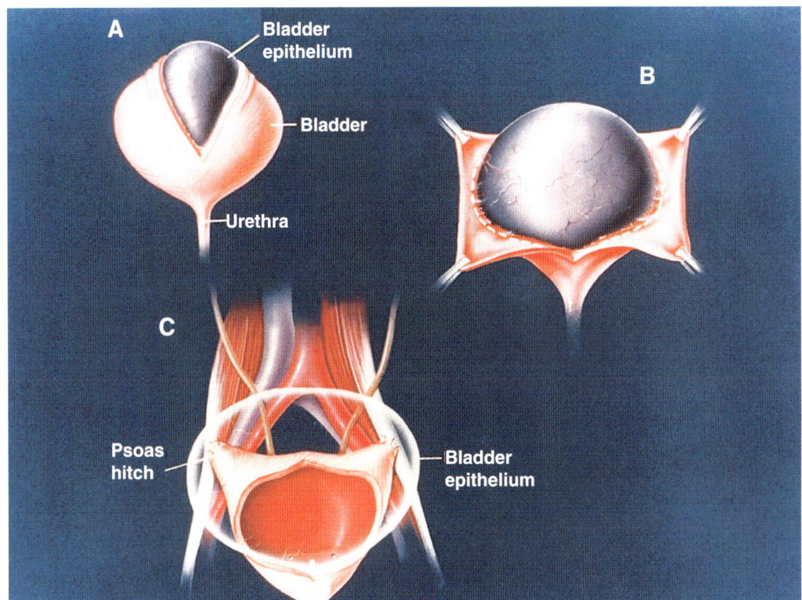

Plate 4 *Diagram of autoaugmentation: (A) detrusor incised, (B) detrusor dissected away from intact urothelium, (C) urothelial bulge with filling.*

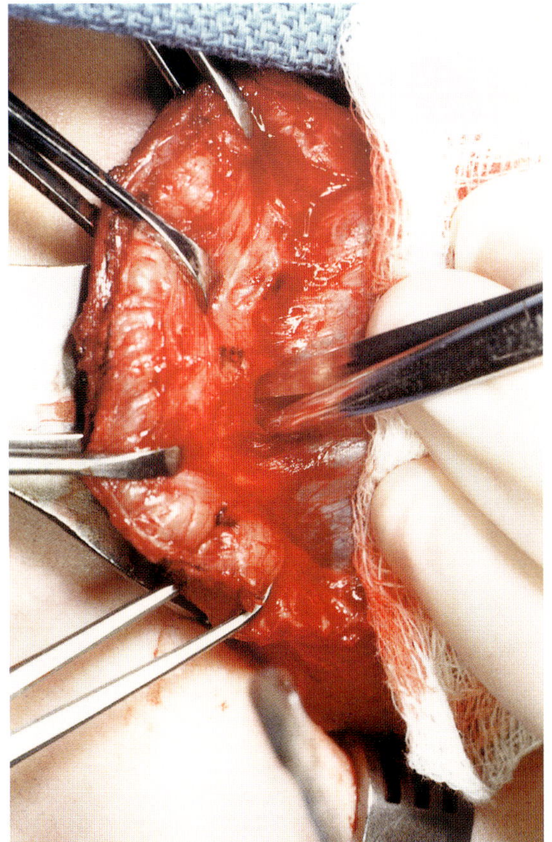

Plate 5 *Urothelium begins to bulge as detrusor is divided.*

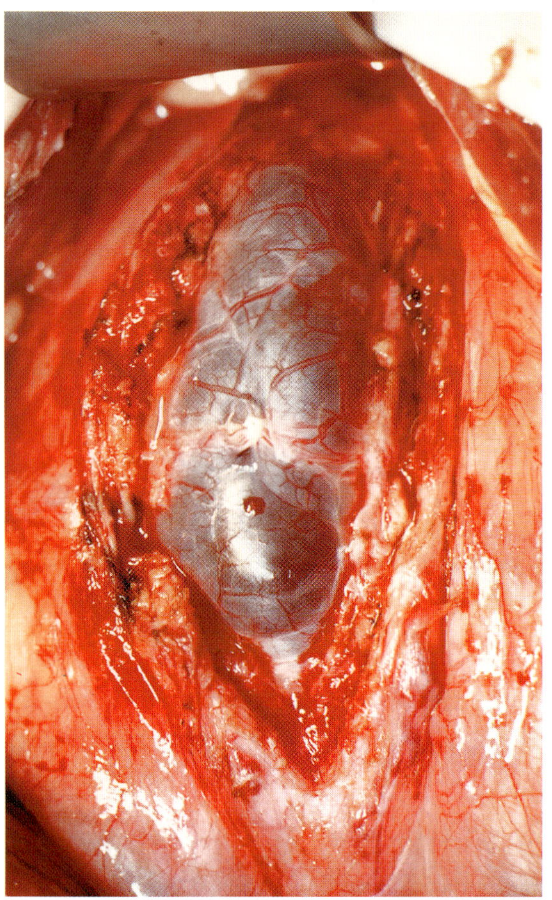

Plate 6 *An Allis clamp retracting laterally on the detrusor edge and gentle finger counteraction over the urothelium expose the plane of dissection.*

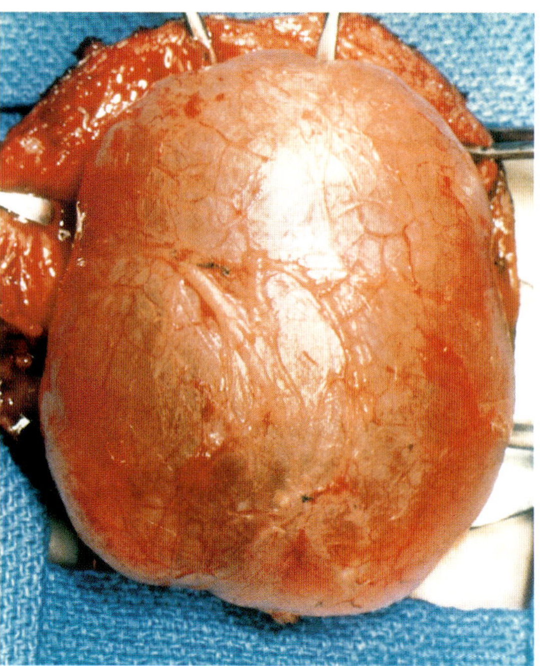

Plate 7 *Urothelial bulge ('diverticulum') at completion.*

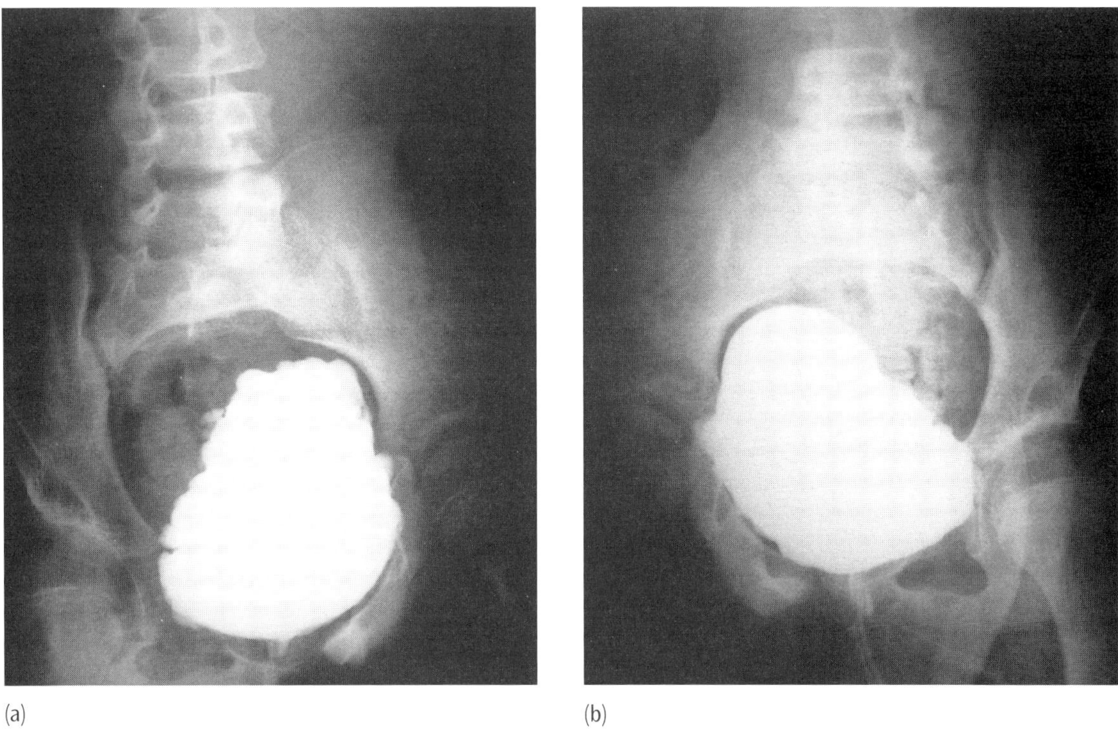

(a) (b)

Figure 10.2 *A patient with myelomeningocele who shows minor compliance improvement from preoperative (a) to postoperative (b) state. This was inadequate to achieve continence.*

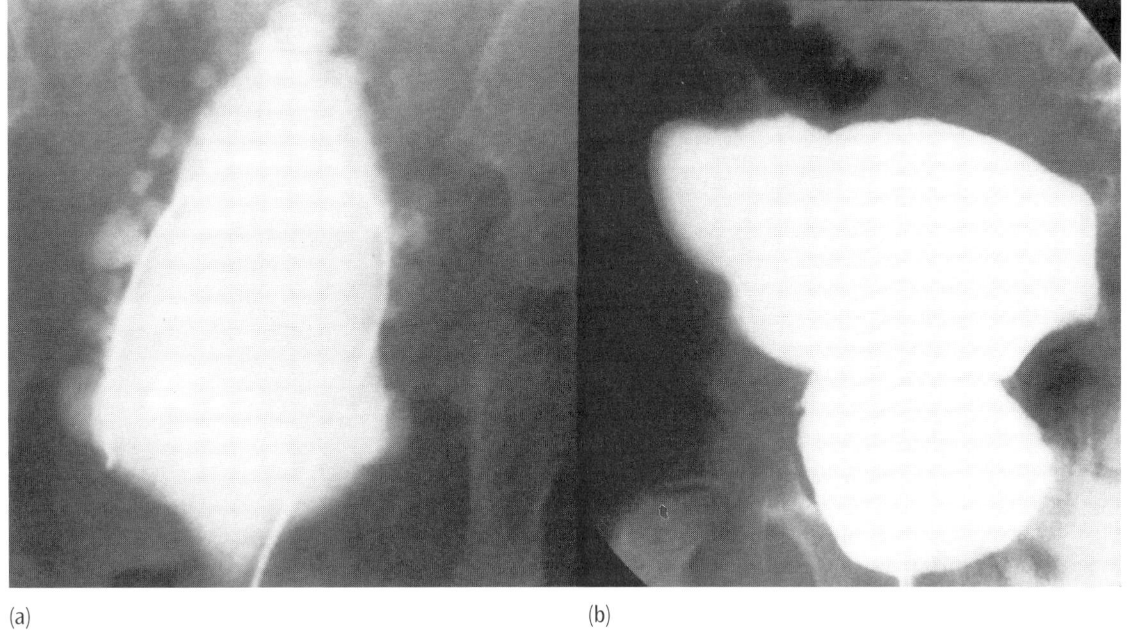

(a) (b)

Figure 10.3 *Pre (a) and post (b) cystograms in a 12-year-old myelomeningocele patient with dramatic improvement after autoaugmentation.*

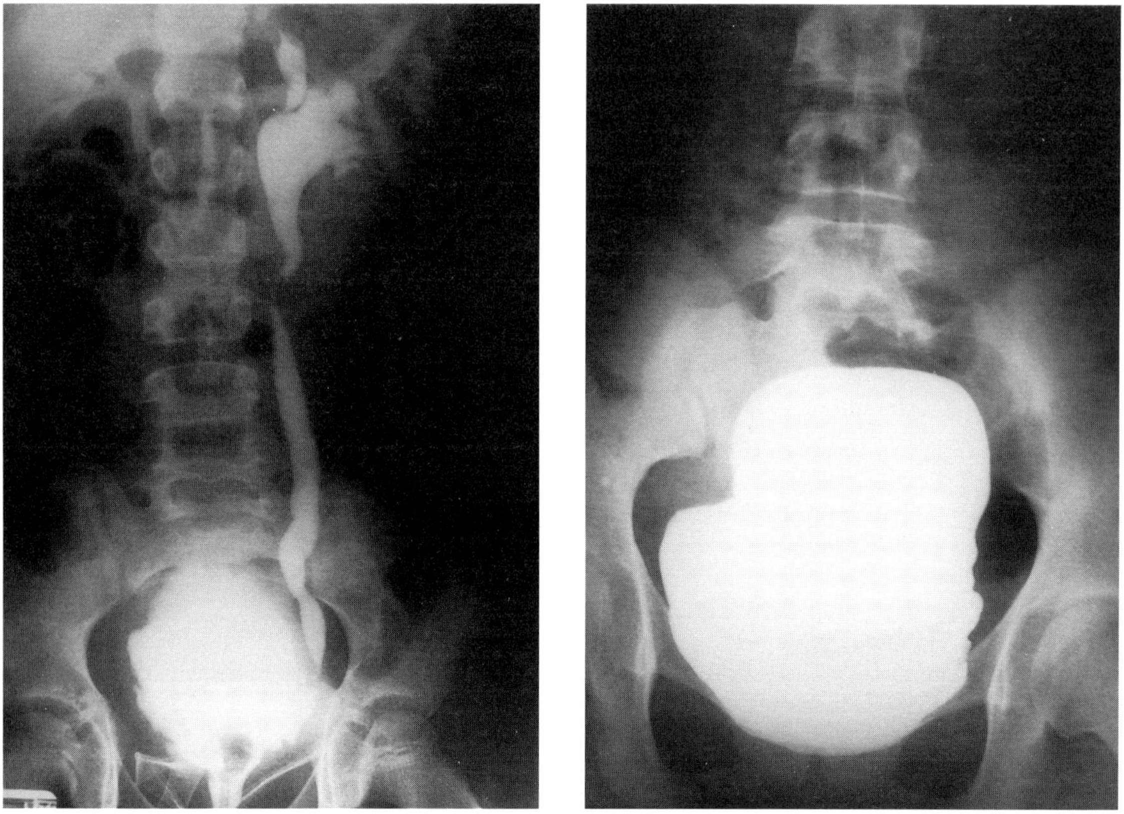

(a) (b)

Figure 10.4 *Preoperative (a) and postoperative five years later: (b) films of a patient with an excellent clinical course. The 'diverticulum' appears to have grown with the patient.*

Clinical outcomes have been encouraging in some, but unpredictable; sample radiographic results are displayed in Figs. 10.2 to 10.4. The results in terms of incontinence, need for intermittent catheterization, change in hydroureteronephrosis, and change in hyperreflexia, are depicted in Figs. 10.5 to 10.8. The overall capacity increased in one-third, was unchanged in one-third, and diminished in the final one-third. Changes in compliance are depicted in individual patients, as shown in Fig. 10.2.

We judged the outcome to be good in 14/30 (47%), fair in 7/30 (23%), and poor in 9/30 (30%). Seven patients have gone on to enterocystoplasty, and one to vesicostomy. In general terms, our experience with autoaugmentation in the pediatric population described suggests that it is quite effective at

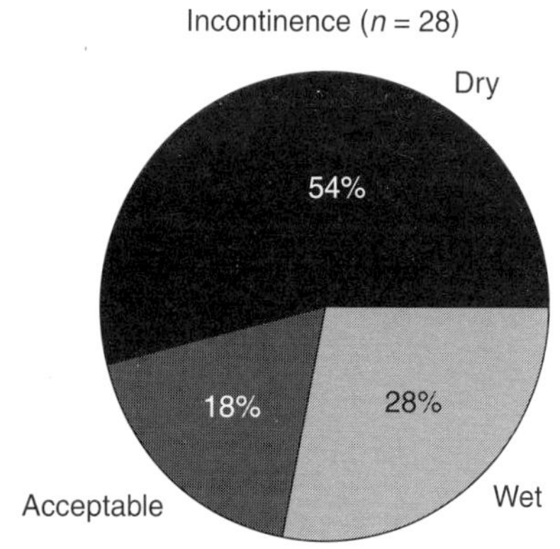

Figure 10.5 *Continence status following autoaugmentation.*

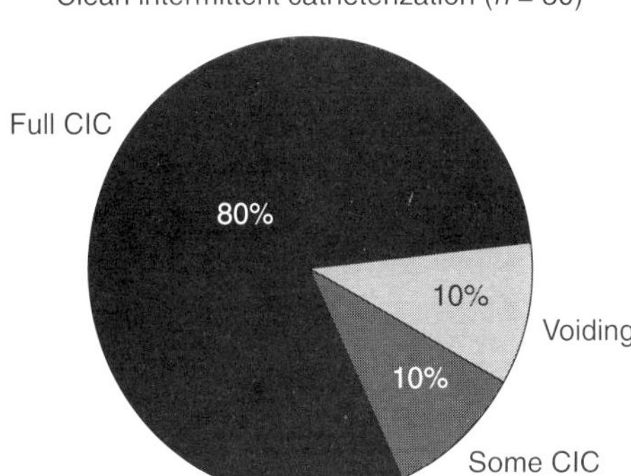

Figure 10.6 *The need for clean intermittent catheterization (CIC) following autoaugmentation.*

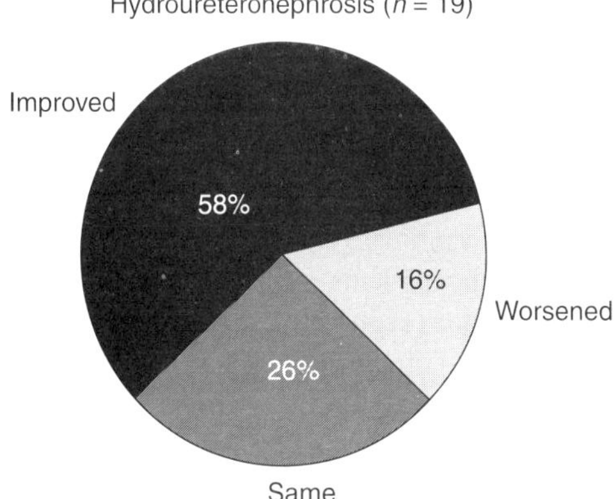

Figure 10.7 *Change in hydroureteronephrosis following autoaugmentation.*

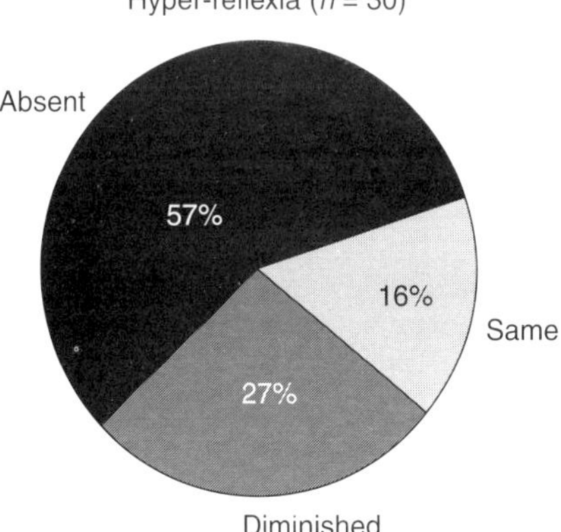

Figure 10.8 *Status of hyperreflexia following autoaugmentation.*

diminishing hyperreflexia, good at improving hydroureteronephrosis and achieving continence, relatively good at improving compliance, and inconsistent in changing maximal bladder capacity. Certainly, the improvement in compliance, as depicted by the volume held at 40 cmH_2O, is largely responsible for the improved hydronephrosis and diminished incontinence (Fig. 10.9).

Elsewhere in the literature there are autoaugmentation experiences of note. Stothers *et al.* reported in 1994 on a series of 12 pediatric patients with neurogenic bladder undergoing the procedure.[15] Improved bladder capacity was found in all patients at 6 months postoperatively, with an average increase of 40% (15–70% range). Interestingly, they also noted a decreased leak-point pressure in many of their patients.

In the first reported series in adults, Kennelly, Gormley, and McGuire described five patients undergoing autoaugmentation for various abnormalities related to poor bladder compliance.[16] They noted a bladder capacity increase between 75 and 310 ml which was a 40–310% increase versus the preoperative capacity. Compliance improved in all, and three of four patients who were preoperatively incontinent regained continence with this procedure alone. Some patients were able to extend the interval between catheterizations, their upper tracts remained stable, and no patient required enterocystoplasty for poor compliance.

In the largest series to date, Stohrer *et al.* reported their experience from a spinal cord injury/disease center in Germany.[17–19] Forty-three patients with various spinal cord pathologies were managed with autoaugmentation. Much more consistent and impressive changes in bladder storage were found than in our pediatric series. Mean bladder capacity went from 121 ml (range 20–300 ml) to 406 ml (range 200–600 ml), while compliance rose from 7.1 ml/cmH_2O (14–30 ml/cmH_2O) to 29.3 ml/cmH_2O (12–62 ml/cmH_2O) (Table 10.1). Stohrer *et al.* judged their results to be: very good, 19; good, eight; improved, one; not improved, two; failures, five and recent surgery, eight.

Further variations on the theme of autoaugmentation have been reported, along with innovative additions to the procedure.[20] This includes creating composite bladders in which demucosalized

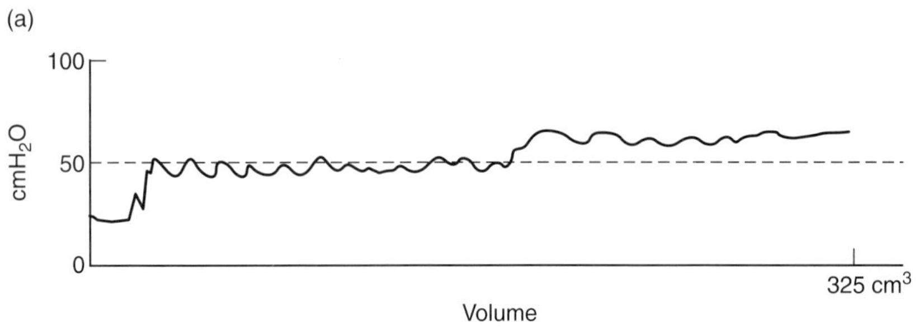

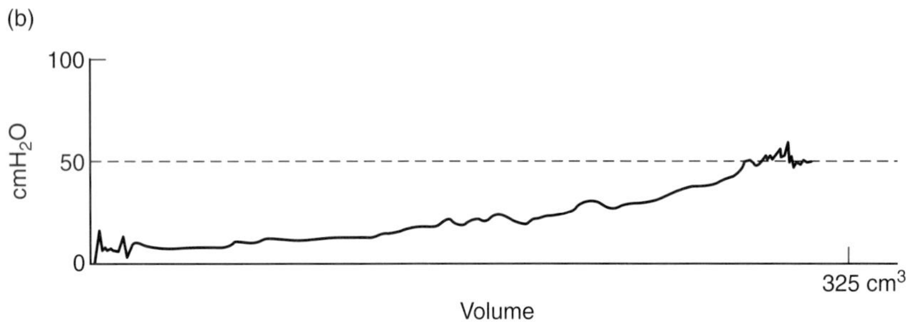

Figure 10.9 *Cystometric tracing in a 7-year-old urethral obstruction patient with little capacity change but a major compliance improvement from preaugmentation (a) to postautoaugmentation (b). This patient gained continence and showed diminished hydronephrosis.*

gastrointestinal segments are added, patched over an autoaugment. The results, potential advantages, and disadvantages of these are addressed in Chapters 11, 12 and 13.

ASSESSMENT AND FUTURE DIRECTIONS

Bladder autoaugmentation has proved technically feasible in the large majority of patients in whom it is undertaken. In the pediatric age group, the results have been unpredictable, as noted.[9,10,13,15] Disappointingly, the success rate has not changed particularly between the first ten, second ten, and final ten patients, despite our attempts to further modify the selection to what we felt were going to be the most appropriate candidates.[13] Other than excluding bladder exstrophy patients as particularly poor candidates, no other preoperative factor was predictive of individual outcome in our pediatric series. It seems likely that there are some intrinsic qualities of the bladder wall, possibly determined by the types of collagen present, the duration and severity of neurogenic change, or other unknown factors which may influence the individual success of the autoaugmentation. These factors may come into play not only with the segment of detrusor removed, but also in determining how remaining detrusor can respond to diminished intravesical pressures postoperatively.

Table 10.1 *Urodynamic data from Stohrer* et al. *on adults undergoing autoaugmentation with at least 6 months follow-up. (Courtesy of Mosby-Yearbook Inc.)*

Parameter	n	Preoperative Average	Standard deviation	Range	Postoperative Average	Standard deviation	Range	p
Bladder capacity (ml)	31	121	74	20–300	406	107	200–600	0.0000
Detrusor voiding pressure (cmH_2O)	32	86.4	52.6	20–280	50.9	25.8	20–130	0.0000
Detrusor compliance (mL/cmH_2O)	32	7.1	6.1	1.4–30	29.3	14.0	12–62	0.0000
Residual urine (ml)	17	21	35	0–130	76	78	0–340	0.0214

Certainly, histologic analysis of the structural components of the bladder wall at the time of autoaugmentation would be of interest. Correlating this to the eventual clinical outcome might allow for better patient selection in the future.

In contrast to the pediatric experience, the adult experience thus far reported is more consistently favorable.[16,19] The majority of patients reported by Stohrer are patients with relatively new-onset neurogenic bladder, secondary to spinal cord injury and disease, and not congenital defects such as myelodysplasia, posterior urethral obstruction, and exstrophy. Review of Stohrer's data indicates that he had a tendency toward early intervention to improve bladder compliance before there is upper tract deterioration,[18] which may also improve the predictability of a successful bladder outcome.

The success in certain of our pediatric patients with bladder autoaugmentation can be very impressive. These patients obtain all the benefits of an augmentation procedure without the significant downside associated with enterocystoplasty. The unpredictability of the eventual result remains a quandary. There seems to be a logical progression toward considering earlier autoaugmentation in patients with neurogenic bladder and urodynamic parameters suggesting a high probability for upper tract deterioration, based on poor bladder compliance. At younger ages, without the long-standing bladder wall changes associated with elevated intravesical pressure, the potential outcome might prove more predictably favorable.

The basic concept of preserving urothelium during bladder augmentation, as occurs with autoaugmentation, appears to be valid. It is our speculation that the augmentation procedure of the future, whether involving preservation of intact urothelium or predicated upon the idea of urothelium growing into a scaffold material (either *in vitro* or *in vivo*), will involve the creation of an augmentation lined with urothelium.

REFERENCES

1. Elder, J.S., Snyder, H.M., Hulbert, W.C. *et al.* (1988) Perforation of the augmented bladder in patients undergoing clean intermittent catheterization. *Journal of Urology,* **140**, 1159–63.
2. Filmer, R. and Spencer, J.R. (1990) Malignancies in bladder augmentations and intestinal conduits. *Journal of Urology,* **143**, 671–8.
3. Hensle, T.W. and Dean, G.E. (1991) Complications of urinary tract reconstruction. *Urologic Clinics of North America,* **18**(4), 755–64.
4. Kelami, A., Dustmann, H.O., Ludtke-Handjery, A. *et al.* (1970) Experimental investigations of bladder regeneration using Teflon felt as bladder wall substitute. *Journal of Urology,* **104,** 693–8.
5. Goldstein, M.D. and Dearden, L.C. (1966) Histology of omentoplasty of the urinary bladder in the rabbit. *Investigative Urology,* **3,** 460–6.
6. Novic, A.C., Straffon, R.A., Banowsky, L.H. *et al.* (1977) Experimental bladder substitution using biodegradable graft of natural tissue. *Urology,* **10**, 118–27.
7. Fishman, I.J., Flores, F.N., Scott, F.B. *et al.* (1987) Use of fresh placental membranes for bladder reconstruction. *Journal of Urology,* **138**, 1291–4.
8. Weingarten, J.L., Paty, R.J. and Cromie, W.J. (1988) Augmentation myoperitoneocystoplasty. *Journal of Urology,* **139**, 131.
9. Cartwright, P.C. and Snow, B.W. (1989) Bladder autoaugmentation: partial detrusor excision to augment the bladder without use of bowel. *Journal of Urology,* **142**, 1050–3.
10. Cartwright, P.C. and Snow, B.W. (1989) Bladder autoaugmentation: early clinical experience. *Journal of Urology,* **142,** 505–8.
11. Johnson, H.W., Nigro, M.K., Stother, L. *et al.* (1994) Laboratory variables of bladder autoaugmentation in an animal model. *Urology,* **44**(2), 260–3.
12. Dewan, P.A., Stefanek, W., Lorenz, C. *et al.* (1994) Autoaugmentation omentocystoplasty in a sheep model. *Urology,* **43**(6), 888–91.
13. Cartwright, P.C. and Snow, B.W. (1995) Bladder autoaugmentation. *Advances in Urology,* Vol. 8. Chicago, Mosby-Year Book.
14. Landa, H.M. and Moorhead, J.D. (1991) Augmentation enterocystoplasty: problems and alternatives. *Dialogues in Pediatric Urology,* **14**, 1–6.
15. Stothers, L., Johnson, H.W., Arnold, W. *et al.* (1994) Bladder autoaugmentation by vesicomyotomy in the pediatric neurogenic bladder. *Urology,* **44**(1), 110–13.

16. Kennelly, M.J., Gormley, E.A. and McGuire, E.J. (1994) Early clinical experience with adult bladder autoaugmentation. *Journal of Urology,* **152**, 303–6.
17. Stohrer, M., Kramer, A., Goepel, M. *et al.* (1995) Bladder autoaugmentation: an alternative for entero-cystoplasty. *Neurourology Urodynamics,* **14,** 11–23.
18. Stohrer, M., Kramer, G., Goepel, M. *et al.* (1997) Partial excision of detrusor muscle (bladder autoaugmentation). In *Patients with Neurogenic Bladder Diseases, Advances in Urology*, Vol. 10. Chicago, Mosby-Yearbook.
19. McDougall, E.M., Clayman, R.V., Figenshau, R.S. *et al.* (1995) Laparoscopic retropubic autoaugmentation of the bladder. *Journal of Urology,* **153**, 123–6.
20. Britansky, R.G., Poppas, D.P., Shichman, S.N. *et al.* (1995) Laparoscopic laser-assisted bladder autoaugmentation. *Urology*, **46**, 31–5

11

Autoaugmentation gastrocystoplasty

PADDY DEWAN

INTRODUCTION

Autoaugmentation gastrocystoplasty (AAGC) has been developed from a combination of the principles of autoaugmentation,[1,2] demucosalized enterocystoplasty,[3–6] and the demonstrated availability of the stomach for bladder augmentation.[7–9] The aim is to achieve a urothelial-lined, augmented bladder.

The principal advantage of a urothelial-lined bladder is the avoidance of the complications of bowel mucosa in contact with urine, which include malignancy,[10,11] mucus and stone formation,[12] metabolic acidosis,[13] and reduced linear growth in children.[14] Unfortunately, the use of gastric-mucosa-lined stomach, as first demonstrated by Sinaiko in 1956[15] and later used for bladder enlargement in both dogs[8] and humans,[16,17] has not been complication free:[18] incorporation of stomach into the bladder adds the risk of the hematuria–dysuria syndrome, metabolic alkalosis, and hypergastrinemia, as mentioned in Chapters 6 and 7.[19–23]

Mau was the first to use the combination of autoaugmentation and enterocystoplasty during a reinnervation experiment in pigs.[24] It would appear that the provision of a muscular backing to the autoaugmentation and, conversely, the full-thickness graft of urothelium onto the denuded intestinal muscle, improve the prospect of producing an enlarged urothelial-lined reservoir. This chapter details a series of experiments which led to the development of the AAGC.

LABORATORY STUDIES

Our first study investigated the feasibility of the AAGC procedure.[25] Ten lambs had a wedge of the greater curve of their fourth stomach mobilized on the right gastroepiploic vessels, and the remainder of the stomach was closed. The mucosa was resected from the isolated segment using cautery. The bladder was then prepared by partly separating the bladder muscle from the urothelium via a midline incision extending from the anterior to the posterior bladder neck, creating the autoaugmentation. The gastric muscle flap was then sutured to the free edge of the bladder muscle with the denuded inner surface of the gastric flap in contact with the urothelial submucosa. These animals were culled at times which allowed review of the survival of the urothelium and the state of inflammation of the neobladder. Histological assessment after augmentation, and subsequent urodynamic and histological studies on other animals, showed survival of the urothelium, rather than death and ingrowth from the adjacent normal bladder. The initial inflammatory infiltrate, which extended into the subepithelial connective tissue, became quiescent and was seen adjacent to otherwise normal transitional epithelium lining the gastric smooth muscle patch.[25]

Follow-up studies compared the normal sheep bladder at 6 and 12 months with bladders subjected to either an AAGC or a clam demucosalized gastrocystoplasty (DMGC).[26] The latter group was added to ensure that autoaugmentation is a necessary part of a successful combined operation. Twenty male lambs had an AAGC and 11 animals underwent a DMGC. The groups were compared with control animals for the radiological, histological, and functional outcomes: urodynamic studies were performed using a double lumen suprapubic catheter.[27] The average bladder volume for the AAGC group at 12 months was greater than that of the control group (401±120 ml vs. 205±77 ml); the demucosalized clam bladders had been less effectively enlarged (286±77 ml). The compliance values for AAGC animals were 14.7±11.3 ml/cmH_2O compared to 9.0±4.8 ml/cmH_2O in the DMGC group, and 9.1±3.7 ml/cmH_2O for the control animals. These animals demonstrated that the autoaugmentation improved the outcome for bladder augmentation using demucosalized stomach.[26]

A further study was then conducted to assess whether autoaugmentation alone would be adequate. Ten male lambs underwent autoaugmentation omentocystoplasty and eight were subsequently studied at 7, 56, and 112 days, and five animals had a urodynamic study at 6 months and four had a repeat study at 12 months.[28,29] In all ten animals the bladder was small and irregular at 10 days, but appeared improved on an intravenous pyelogram at 3 weeks. In the five animals that underwent a urodynamic study at 6 months, the bladder was found to be relatively small compared to the control group. Histologically, survival of the urothelium and subepithelial connective tissue layers was noted at 7 days and marked inflammation, prominent fibrosis, and even metaplastic bone formation were seen subsequently. In other words, autoaugmentation did not enlarge the sheep bladder.[28,29]

CLINICAL APPLICATION

Autoaugmentation gastrocystoplasty was first applied clinically, only after the successful outcome in sheep, and has been used in ten children with a neurogenic bladder. Urodynamic studies were performed preoperatively to confirm the presence of a high-pressure bladder in children presenting with urinary incontinence and renal compromise, despite clean intermittent catheterization and anticholinergic therapy. The gastric segment was used as the source of muscle in the initial cases, because of its availability and because of the greater success using stomach, than colon, in the sheep.

OPERATIVE TECHNIQUE (Fig. 11.1)

A long midline abdominal incision was made and the adequacy of the length of the right gastroepiploic arcade checked. The right gastroepiploic branches to the greater curve of the stomach and duodenum were divided up to the medial end of the anticipated gastric patch. A wedge segment of the stomach was clamped, incised, and separated from the remainder of the stomach, which was closed with a continuous polyglycolic acid suture. The gastric mucosa was removed from the isolated segment of muscle using diathermy dissection, taking care to protect the underlying muscle, while avoiding retained islands of gastric mucosa. This was achieved by cautery dissection, which removed the muscularis mucosae and part of the submucosal layer from the underlying gastric muscle. The bladder was then prepared by first incising the detrusor in the midline, from the anterior to the posterior bladder neck region. The detrusor was separated from the urothelium through the submucal plane for approximately one-third of

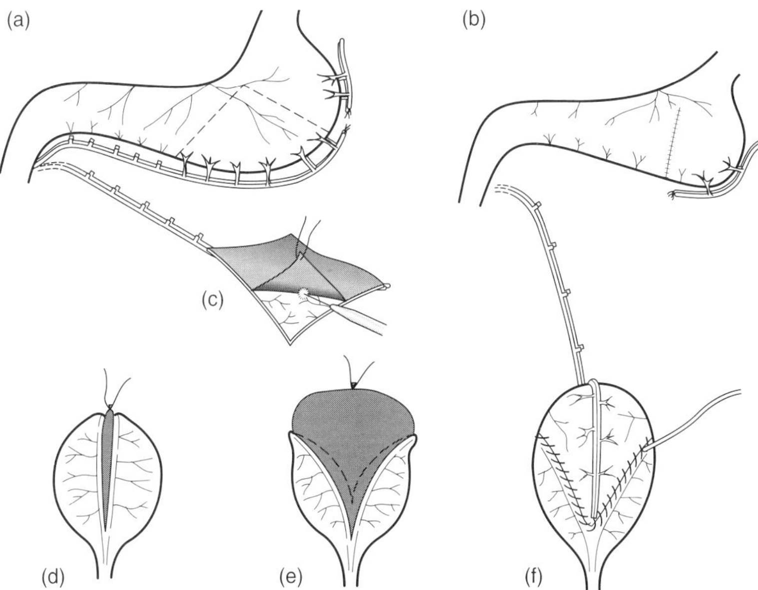

Figure 11.1 *The principal steps in the operation of autoaugmentation gastrocystoplasty. (a) A wedged-shaped segment of the greater curve is mobilized on a vascular pedicle of the right gastroepiploic vessels. (b) The stomach is closed by continuous suture and the pedicle mobilized more proximally if required. (c) The mucosa is removed from the gastric patch by diathermy dissection. (d) A stay suture is placed in the dome of the bladder, and the muscle and mucosa of the bladder are separated by sharp dissection. (e) The bladder layers are separated until a large, wide-mouth diverticulum is created. (f) The denuded gastric patch surface is laid over the submucosal layer of the bladder and sutured in place. Reproduced with permission of Springer International from Lorenz, C. and Dewan, P.A. (1993) The evolution of augmentation gastrocystoplasty.* Pediatric Surgery International, **8**, 491–5.

the bladder muscle. The resulting herniation of the bladder mucosa was then covered with the demucosalized inner surface of the gastric patch. The urachal remnant was sutured to the midpoint of the gastric muscle flap, which was then sutured edge-to-edge with the bladder muscle. The bladder mucosa was, therefore, left intact, covered with both bladder and stomach muscle. The bladder was drained via a urethral catheter for 10 days, with the catheter bag being suspended 15 cm above the bladder after the first 12 hours, to encourage adherence of the urothelium to the stomach segment.

RESULTS

Microscopic examination of the discarded gastric mucosa indicated that both the muscularis mucosae and at least part of the submucosa were removed from all seromuscular flaps. Furthermore, no mucus was seen in any of the specimens of urine examined histologically postoperatively. Five patients have subsequently had open or cystoscopic inspection of the bladder, none of whom has shown any evidence of gastric mucosa regrowth. The urodynamic and continence results are shown in Table 11.1.

DISCUSSION

Bladder augmentation protects kidneys and improves urinary continence in a range of primary and secondary causes of bladder dysfunction. However, most of these patients are kept dry with intermittent catheterization[30] and anticholinergic medication. Those with ongoing renal deterioration,

Table 11.1 *The urodynamic results for the ten patients who have had an autoaugmentation gastrocystoplasty. The preoperative and postoperative volumes and compliance are given*

Patient	Volumes (ml)		Compliance (ml/cmH_2O)		Follow-up (months)	
	Pre	Post	Pre	Post		
1	50	460	1.0	35.0	27	Dry
2	50	412	1.0	25.9	39	Dry
3	80	321	1.0	40.0	26	Dry
4	90	208	1.0	15.5	25	Dry
5	70	477	–	34.6	17	Dry
6	20	280	<1.0	10.8	10	Wet – poor CIC
7	50	263	<1.0	11.0	32	Dry
8	50	250	<1.0	10.1	12	Dry
9	50	310	<1.0	30.1	24	Ileocystoplasty
10	150	315	2.5	6.3	12	Dry

despite frequent bladder drainage, need bladder augmentation, which is currently most often achieved with full-thickness small bowel or colon.

The alternative procedures, which aim to achieve a urothelial-lined bladder, can use muscle from the gastrointestinal tract. The formation of a urothelial-lined, bowel-muscle-augmented bladder was initially pioneered by Shoemaker in 1955.[4] A number of studies in the dog, calf, rat, and pig have subsequently used demucosalized segments of intestine for enterocystoplasty.[6,24,31–6] In these studies the raw enteric patch was covered by the ingrowth of urothelium from the adjacent bladder, a technique which works well in small animals[35] but is less satisfactory when a larger area is to be covered, as in larger animals; the larger the bladder, the greater the area to be resurfaced and the more extensive the scarring before the muscle is lined by urothelium. This was again shown in our work with demucosalized stomach and colon, particularly by the demucosalized gastric muscle lined by an autoaugmentation, an operation which improves the urodynamic results compared to demucosalized clam gastrocystoplasty without autoaugmentation.[26] Notably, electrolyte absorption patterns for the urothelial-lined gut muscle are the same as for the normal bladder.[33]

Obviously, methods which utilize seromuscular bowel segments require consideration of the technique of demucosalization so as to prevent fibrotic changes and enteric mucosal regrowth:[3–5,34,37–41] removal of the muscularis mucosae has been associated with contracture and calcification in the large and small bowel flaps.[4,38,40,41] However, when Motley *et al.*[34] preserved the submucosa, contraction of the patch still occurred; Buson *et al.*[38] failed to produce any significant bladder augmentation in an autoaugmentation colocystoplasty (AACC) model with the submucosa and muscularis mucosae specifically undisturbed; and Cheng *et al.*[42] found fibrosis and contraction of reversed distal ileum from which no mucosa had been removed. We also found poor urodynamic results when the muscularis mucosae and submucosa were preserved in our AACC and DMGC animals.[43] Overall, it would appear that contact of the enteric segment with urine is the main cause of the contraction of the gut segment, not whether the submucosa is left *in situ*. Autoaugmentation appears to provide an immediate lining which reduces the inflammation in the augmentation patch, at least when sheep stomach and dog colon are used.[40,44] The advantage of the removal of the muscularis mucosae, and most of the submucosa, is the greater reliability of preventing enteric mucosal regrowth. Shoemaker, when he retained the submucosa and, therefore, the muscularis mucosae, demonstrated regrowth of ileal mucosa in all animals.[4] Blandy removed both the submucosa and mucosa from ileal flaps, thus preventing ileal mucosa regrowth.[37] Subsequent animal studies support our finding that failure to specifically remove the muscularis mucosae results in mucosal regrowth.[34,38,40,41,45] In our study, colonic mucosal regrowth was seen in four of five animals undergoing demucosalized colocystoplasty

(DMCC), all of which had preservation of the muscularis mucosae and submucosa: all our sheep, in which the muscularis mucosae and part of the submucosa were removed, showed no regrowth.[46] Enteric mucosal regrowth has also been attributed to early and later contact of the inner layer of the seromuscular patch with urothelium, a conclusion negated by the finding of enteric mucosal regeneration both with reversed flaps placed over an autoaugmentation and when enteric flaps are added to the opened bladder.[41,45]

Autoaugmentation, popularized by Cartwright and Snow,[1,2] makes use of the ability to separate the muscular and mucosal layers of the bladder, as experienced with ureteric reimplants and bladder mucosal grafts for hypospadias repair. The technique can consist of excision of the detrusor[1,47]or peeling the muscle from part of the underlying mucosa;[48] we have tended to use the latter, recognizing that the different approaches have never been studied comparatively. Survival of the mucosa, as seen in the omental, gastric, and colonic patch animals in our studies, is predicted by fluorescent angiography studies, which confirm mucosal blood flow.[49]

Sheep bladders which had undergone autoaugmentation were shown in our studies to be urodynamically unsatisfactory when compared to the controls.[28,29] This contrasts to the results seen in the Cartwright and Snow dog experiments, in which the animals were sacrificed early, perhaps before a significant degree of the progressive fibrosis had occurred. Improved results are indeed obtained if the autoaugmentation is given gastric muscular backing, results that seem to improve the later after the operation the studies are conducted.[26] The stomach has been chosen as the donor site because of the compliant nature of gastric muscle and the ease of separation of the mucosa and muscle.

However, when the AAGC was applied to patients, transient weight gain problems were seen in two of our patients[50] and were reported by Gold *et al.* when they used stomach for bladder augmentation in children.[51] Therefore, patients are offered an AACC, provided that the dissection of the mucosa from the colon muscle could be achieved, as judged from the progress of the demucosalization in its initial stages. The use of colon was motivated by a patient who was underweight for age, the success in the pig and the dog autoaugmentation colocystoplasty,[40,44] and the greater ease of removal of the human colonic mucosa than that of the sheep.[52] Autoaugmentation colocystoplasty was used in spite of the unsuccessful results in the sheep study and a number of animal studies that had shown mucosal regrowth with large and small bowel demucosalized enterocystoplasty.[6,34] The adverse results were discounted because it was felt that a combination of the delicate nature of the sheep colon with the difficulty and trauma of demucosalization may have mitigated against success of the urothelial colocystoplasty, preventing the underlying autoaugmentation from providing any outcome advantage. Also, removal of part of the submucosa in children has proven to give the same protection against enteric mucosal regrowth as suggested from laboratory studies.[52]

We found favorable urodynamic results in the majority of our patients undergoing autoaugmentation enterocystoplasty, using either stomach or colon, when the muscularis mucosae and part of the submucosa were removed. Likewise, Nguyen *et al.*[53] reported improved bladder capacity and compliance in 11 patients undergoing demucosalized augmentation gastrocystoplasty. At postoperative cystoscopy, two of their patients demonstrated bladders in which the native and augmented portions were largely indistinguishable, with no evidence of gastric mucosal regrowth. Although the urodynamic findings are not as impressive as for routine enterocystoplasty, not all enteric-mucosa-lined enterocystoplasties achieve an adequate result. Kockelberger *et al.*[54] and Smith *et al.*[55] recorded poor capacity increases; Sidi *et al.*[56] have indicated the need for ongoing anticholinergic medication; and urinary diversion has been required in some patients.[54] Furthermore, Cher and Allen reported seven children between the ages of 6 and 14 years with a routine enterocystoplasty who had an average postaugmentation volume of only 100 ml and an average compliance of 2.9 ml/cmH_2O; volumes as low as 50 ml and compliance values down to 1.0 ml/cmH_2O were reported.[57]

The major advantage of autoaugmentation demucosalized enterocystoplasty is the avoidance of the long-term complications of incorporation of gastrointestinal tract epithelium into the urinary tract. However, the operative time and the technical difficulty are both greater than for a routine clam enterocystoplasty. In those at risk of fecal incontinence if their colon length is reduced, the best source of muscle would seem to be the stomach; if intolerance of adequate meals may be a significant problem after an AAGC, a demucosalized colon with autoaugmentation would be the author's preferred option.

REFERENCES

1. Cartwright, P.C. and Snow, B.W. (1989) Bladder autoaugmentation: early clinical experience. *Journal of Urology,* **142**, 505–8.
2. Cartwright, P.C. and Snow, B.W. (1989) Bladder autoaugmentation: partial detrusor excision to augment the bladder without use of bowel. *Journal of Urology,* **142**, 1050–3.
3. Blandy, J.P. (1964) The feasibility of preparing an ideal substitute for the urinary bladder. *Annals of the Royal College of Surgeons of England,* **35,** 287–311.
4. Shoemaker, W.C. (1955) Reversed seromuscular grafts in urinary tract reconstruction. *Journal of Urology,* **74,** 453–75.
5. Shoemaker, W.C., Bower, R. and Long, D.M. (1957) A new technique for bladder reconstruction. *Surgery, Gynecology and Obstetrics,* **105,** 645–50.
6. Shoemaker, W.C. and Maracci, H. (1955) The experimental use of seromuscular grafts in bladder reconstruction. *Journal of Urology,* **73,** 314–21.
7. Adams, M.C., Mitchell, M.E. and Rink, R.C. (1988) Gastrocystoplasty: an alternative solution to the problem of urological reconstruction in the severely compromised patient. *Journal of Urology,* **140,** 1152–6.
8. Leong, C.H. and Ong, G.B. (1972) Gastrocystoplasty in dogs. *Australian and New Zealand Journal of Surgery,* **41,** 272–9.
9. Sinaiko, E.S. (1960) Artificial bladder from gastric pouch. *Surgery, Gynecology and Obstetrics,* **111,** 155–62.
10. Filmer, R.B. and Spencer, J.R. (1990) Malignancies in bladder augmentations and intestinal conduits. *Journal of Urology,* **143,** 671–8.
11. Kälble, T., Amelung, F., Busse, K. *et al.* (1994) Prophylaxis of carcinomas following urinary diversion by surgical methods. *Journal of Urology,* **151** (Suppl.), 500A.
12. Blyth, B., Ewalt, D.H., Duckett, J.W. *et al.* (1992) Lithogenic properties of enterocystoplasty. *Journal of Urology,* **148,** 575–7.
13. Nurse, D.E. and Mundy, A.R. (1989) Metabolic complications of cystoplasty. *British Journal of Urology,* **63,** 165–70.
14. Wagstaff, K.E., Woodhouse, C.R.J., Duffy, P.G. *et al.* (1992) Delayed linear growth in children with enterocystoplasties. *British Journal of Urology,* **69,** 314–17.
15. Sinaiko, E. (1956) Artificial bladder from segment of stomach and study of effect of urine on gastric secretion. *Surgery, Gynecology and Obstetrics,* **102,** 433–8.
16. Leong, C.H. (1978) Use of the stomach for bladder replacement and urinary diversion. *Annals of the Royal College of Surgeons of England,* **60,** 283–9.
17. Piser, J.A., Mitchell, M.E., Kulb, T.B. *et al.* (1987) Gastrocystoplasty and colocystoplasty in canines: the metabolic consequences of acute saline and acid loading. *Journal of Urology,* **138,** 1009–13.
18. Klee, L.W., Hoover, D.M., Mitchell, M.E. *et al.* (1990) Long-term effects of gastrocystoplasty in rats. *Journal of Urology,* **144,** 1283–7.
19. Castro-Diaz, D., Froemming, C., Manival, J.C. *et al.* (1992) The influence of urinary diversion on experimental gastrocystoplasty. *Journal of Urology,* **148**, 571–4.
20. Gosalbez, R. Jr, Woodard, J.R., Broecker, B.H. *et al.* (1993) Metabolic complications of the use of stomach for urinary reconstruction. *Journal of Urology,* **150,** 710–12.
21. Kinahan, T.J., Khoury, A.E., McLorie, GA. *et al.* (1992) Omeprazole in post-gastrocystoplasty metabolic alkalosis and aciduria. *Journal of Urology,* **147,** 435–7.
22. Muraishi, O., Ikado, S., Yamashita, T. *et al.* (1992) Gastrocystoplasty in dogs: an ulcerating effect of acid urine. *Journal of Urology,* **147,** 242–5.
23. Nguyen, D.H., Bain, M.A., Salmonson, K.L. *et al.* (1993) The syndrome of dysuria and hematuria in pediatric urinary reconstruction with stomach. *Journal of Urology,* **150,** 707–9.
24. Mau, H. (1980) Die neurogene Blase – tierexperimentelle Untersuchungen zur Restauration der Blasenfunktion,

Habilitationsschrift, Humboldt-Universität zu Berlin, pp. 1–300.
25. Dewan, P.A. and Byard, R.W. (1993) Autoaugmentation gastrocystoplasty in a sheep model. *British Journal of Urology,* **72,** 56–9.
26. Dewan, P.A., Stefanek, W., Lorenz, C., *et al.* (1995) Autoaugmentation gastrocystoplasty and demucosalised gastrocystoplasty in a sheep model. *Urology,* **45**, 291–5.
27. Dewan, P.A. (1995) A double lumen suprapubic urodynamic catheter. *Australian and New Zealand Journal of Surgery,* **65,** 672–3.
28. Dewan, P.A., Owen, A.J., Stefanek, W. *et al.* (1995) Late follow-up of autoaugmentation omentocystoplasty in a sheep model. *Australian and New Zealand Journal of Surgery,* **65,** 596–9.
29. Dewan, P.A., Stefanek, W., Lorenz, C. *et al.* (1994) Autoaugmentation omentocystoplasty in a sheep model. *Urology,* **43,** 888–91.
30. Lapides, J., Diokno, A.C., Silber, S.J. *et al.* (1972) Clean, intermittent self-catheterization in the treatment of urinary tract disease. *Journal of Urology,* **107,** 458–61.
31. Badiola de, F., Manivel, J.C. and Gonzalez, R. (1991) Seromuscular enterocystoplasty in rats. *Journal of Urology,* **146,** 559–62.
32. Blandy, J.P. and McDonald, J.H. (1961) Heterotopic ossification in uroepithelial regeneration on grafts of ileum and colon. *Surgery for Urology,* **12,** 498–500.
33. Grotzinger, P.J., Shoemaker, W.C., Ulin, A.W., Marucci, H.D. and Martin, W.L. (1954) The use of inverted seromuscular grafts from the ileum and colon for reconstruction of the urinary bladder. *Annals of Surgery,* **140,** 832–8.
34. Motley, R.C., Montgomery, B.T., Zollman, P.E. *et al.* (1990) Augmentation cystoplasty utilizing de-epithelialized sigmoid colon: a preliminary study. *Journal of Urology,* **143,** 1257–60.
35. Oesch, I. (1988) Neourothelium in bladder augmentation. *European Journal of Urology,* **14,** 328–9.
36. Pippi Salle, J.L., Fraga, J.C.S., Lucid, A. *et al.* (1990) Seromuscular enterocystoplasty in dogs. *Journal of Urology,* **144,** 454–6.
37. Blandy, J.P. (1961) Ileal pouch with transitional epithelium and anal sphincter as a continent urinary reservoir. *Journal of Urology,* **86,** 749–67.
38. Buson, H., Manivel, J.C., Dayanç, M. *et al.* (1994) Seromuscular colocystoplasty lined with urothelium (SCLU): experimental study. *Urology,* **44**, 743–8.
39. Garibay, J.T., Manivel, J.C. and Gonzalez, R. (1995) Effect of seromuscular colocystoplasty lined with urothelium and partial detrusorectomy on a new canine model of reduced bladder capacity. *Journal of Urology,* **154,** 903–6.
40. Lima, S.V.C., Araujo, L.A.P., Vilar, F.O. *et al.* (1995) Nonsecretory sigmoid cystoplasty: experimental and clinical results. *Journal of Urology,* **153,** 1651–4.
41. Lutz, N. and Frey, P. (1995) Enterocystoplasty using modified pedicled, detubularised, de-epithelialised sigmoid patches in the mini-pig model. *Journal of Urology.* **154,** 893–8.
42. Cheng, E., Rento, R., Grayhack, J.T. *et al.* (1995) Reversed seromuscular flaps in the urinary tract in dogs. *Journal of Urology,* **152**, 2252–7.
43. Dewan, P.A., Lorenz, C., Stefanek, W. *et al.* (1994) Urothelial lined colocystoplasty in a sheep model. *European Journal of Urology,* **26,** 240–6.
44. Garibay, J.T. and Gonzalez, R. (1995) Effect of seromuscular colocystoplasty lined with urothelium (SCLU) and simple detrusorectomy in a canine model of reduced bladder capacity. *Journal of Urology,* **153,** 339A.
45. Gonzalez, R., Buson, H., Reid, C. *et al.* (1995) Seromuscular colocystoplasty lined with urothelium: experience with 16 patients. *Urology,* **45,** 124–9.
46. Dewan, P.A., Close, C.E., Byard, R.W. *et al.* (1997) Enteric mucosal regrowth after bladder augmentation using demucosalised gut segments. *Journal of Urology,* **158**, 1141–6.
47. Moorhead, J.D. (1991) Detrusorectomy: autoaugmentation by a different name. *Dialogues of Pediatric Urology,* **14,** 4–5.
48. Gordon, E., Malone, P.R., Duffy, P.G. *et al.* (1991) The place of autocystoplasty in the management of the neuropathic bladder. (Abstract.) *British Journal of Urology,* **68,** 644.
49. Snow, B.W. and Cartwright, M.D. (1991) Bladder augmentation. In King, L.R., Stone, A.R. and Webster, G.D. (eds.). *Bladder Reconstruction and Continent Urinary Diversion.* Chicago, London, Year Book Medical Publishers: 107–14.

50. Dewan, P.A. and Stefanek, W. (1994) Autoaugmentation gastrocystoplasty: early clinical results. *British Journal of Urology,* **74**, 460–4.
51. Gold, B.D., Bhoopalam, P.S., Reifen, R.M. *et al.* (1992) Gastrointestinal complications of gastrocystoplasty. *Archives of Diseases in Childhood,* **67,** 1272–6.
52. Dewan, P.A. and Stefanek, W. (1994) Autoaugmentation colocystoplasty: a case report. *Pediatric Surgery International,* **9**, 526–8.
53. Nguyen, D.H., Mitchell, M.E., Horowitz, M. *et al.* (1996) Demucosalised augmentation gastrocystoplasty with bladder autoaugmentation in pediatric patients. *Journal of Urology,* **156,** 206–9.
54. Kockelberger. R.C., Tan, J.B.L., Bates, C.B. *et al.* (1991) Clam enterocystoplasty in general urological practice. *British Journal of Urology,* **68,** 38–41.
55. Smith, R.B., Van Cangh, P., Skinner, D.G. *et al.* (1977) Augmentation enterocystoplasty: a critical review. *Journal of Urology,* **118,** 35–9.
56. Sidi, A.A., Aliabadi, H. and Gonzalez, R. (1987) Enterocystoplasty in the management and reconstruction of the pediatric neurogenic bladder. *Journal of Pediatric Surgery,* **22,** 153–7.
57. Cher, M.L. and Allen, T.D. (1993) Continence in the myelodysplastic patient following enterocystoplasty. *Journal of Urology,* **149**, 1103–6.
58. Lorenz, C. and Dewan, P.A. (1993) The evolution of autoaugmentation gastrocystoplasty. *Pediatric Surgery International*, **8**, 491–5.

12

Autoaugmentation colocystoplasty: laboratory research

NICOLAS LUTZ AND PETER FREY

INTRODUCTION

Although many techniques of bladder augmentation have been proposed for the reconstruction of an adequate lower urinary tract, none has gained universal approval, as discussed in Chapter 10. Autoaugmentation is a procedure consisting of detrusorectomy or detrusoromyotomy resulting in a large prolapsing intact urothelium which will increase the volume of the bladder. It was first popularized by Cartwright in 1989,[1] based on the idea of Couvelaire,[2] and produced a urothelial-lined reservoir which avoided the harmful contact of urine with the intestinal mucosa of conventional enterocystoplasties. Unfortunately, the poor mechanical properties of the bulging urothelium, as well as its possible progressive shrinkage, have not given satisfactory long-term urodynamics results.[3–6] In an attempt to overcome this problem, several studies have been performed using pedicled, detubularized and de-epithelialized colonic or gastric segments to further cover, protect, and possibly bring substantial mechanical and nutritional support to the thin urothelial wall.[4,6–16]

The sigmoid colon is surgically easily accessible. It is anatomically close to the bladder and can be mobilized with its well-defined vascular pedicle without affecting colonic function. A long segment can easily be harvested to obtain, once detubularized, a patch which will allow bladder reconstruction to an adequate capacity. Extraperitoneal bladder reconstruction with a sigmoid patch is possible[17] and may be advantageous in case of urinary leakage or perforation.

Today, enterocystoplasty is still one of the most popular bladder augmentation procedures, despite its significant short-term and long-term complications,[18] which are mainly due to the remaining mucus-secreting and acid-absorbing intestinal mucosa. Several studies have been performed to assess the feasibility and outcome of total epithelial removal of intestinal detubularized segments in order to avoid mucus secretion, acid absorption or secondary potential malignant changes of the mucosa.[19–24]

This chapter discusses the latest experimental studies on bladder autoaugmentation covered with a pedicled and de-epithelialized sigmoid patch.[4,6,7,9,25,26]

TECHNIQUE OF DETRUSOR MYOTOMY

The technique of autoaugmentation is based on the idea of removing a retracted or diseased detrusor in order to free an elastic, thin, and intact urothelium which will bulge and increase total bladder capacity and compliance.[1,2] Both detrusor resection above the level of the trigone and simple sagittal detrusor myotomy have been advocated for this purpose.[1,27,28] The procedure is performed on a catheterized bladder, which is filled to normal capacity and dissected with the aid of magnifying glasses or a microscope. Meticulous care must be taken to leave the urothelium intact. We prefer to leave a few muscle fibers over the bulging urothelium rather than to try to free it completely, therefore keeping to a minimum the risk of concomitant urothelial injury and urine leakage. Any tear in the urothelium should be closed, as a leak of urine between the urothelial bulging pouch and the de-epithelialized bowel segment will prevent adhesion and survival of the urothelium and could furthermore cause intramural inflammation and shrinkage of the patch. Closure of a urothelial defect is best achieved by tying the grasped tear with resorbable suture material. Any attempt at suturing the tear may end in more damage and a bigger hole. A sagittal detrusoromyotomy over half the circumference of the bladder is sufficient to obtain a large bulging urothelium and significantly increase total bladder capacity.

Laparoscopic transabdominal or retroperitoneal autoaugmentations have been described with adequate short-term results.[29–31]

TECHNIQUE OF COLONIC PATCH PREPARATION

Although the ileocecal valve has been used for conventional enterocystoplasties in adults,[32] we would not recommend using this intestinal segment in a child, because of its unique and vital absorption of vitamins and biliary acids. On the other hand, the sigmoid colon can easily be isolated from the rest of the digestive tract, with no secondary absorption impairment, once the continuity of the alimentary tract has been re-established.

Detubularization of the colonic segment is always performed on its antimesenteric border. The intestinal patch can then be used with or without reshaping. We, as well as Dewan *et al.*, have not modified the shape of the sigmoid patch before suturing it to the side of the bladder wall because the bulging urothelium being covered, which was obtained following sagittal detrusoromyotomy, had a similar shape.[9,15] Other authors have performed a reconfiguration of the patch as an inverted U, or shaped as a cup,[33] prior to the coverage of urothelium obtained following subtotal detrusoromyectomy.

Care must be taken when choosing the vascular supply of the segment of colon to be used for urothelial coverage. Too short a pedicle will result in unnecessary traction and potential ischemia of the detubularized and de-epithelialized bowel segment. Adequate and consistent blood supply to the patch is vital for the success of the operation. We therefore never clamp the pedicle, although some authors have suggested it to decrease bleeding during de-epithelialization.[25] The direct vision of bleeding vessels on the surface of the patch during de-epithelialization allows precise bipolar cauterization, with no thermic injury to the remaining wall. Unipolar cautery implies high temperature and currents through a narrow vascular pedicle with potential injury to both pedicle and underlying muscle layers, and should therefore be avoided. The bleeding can also be controlled by the application of gauze sponges moistened with an epinephrine solution applied onto the submucosa.[7] Although mechanical intestinal obstruction due to the intraperitoneal position of the pedicle has never reported, we believe that a retroperitoneal position is safer when feasible.

It remains clear that when performing a de-epithelialized enterocystoplasty, meticulous intestinal mucosa removal is of the utmost importance and is dependent on surgical technique as well as on the animal model that is used.

Regarding the problems related to suturing, it is worth mentioning that in their reversed ileal flap technique, Campbell suggested the possibility of intestinal mucosal contamination of the serosa through full-thickness sutures.[19] Nowadays, watertight sutures can be achieved using thin partial-thickness resorbable sutures, as well as clips with or without fibrin glue. Care must be taken not to perforate the bulging urothelium when tying the free edges of the detrusor to the borders of the patch. Nonresorbable sutures are useful to mark the border of the patch when morphometric analysis is to be performed, but should remain out of the bladder lumen in order to avoid the formation of calculi. The CO_2 laser has also been used successfully in the rat for bladder tissue welding and has been found to be significantly faster than conventional microsurgical enterocystoplasty.[34]

Drainage of the space between the urothelial bulging pouch and the de-epithelialized colonic patch does not appear to be necessary, providing that complete and consistent hemostasis of the surface of the patch has been achieved. Furthermore, no organized clot or calcification between the urothelium and colonic muscle was seen at sacrifice in studies where no drainage was carried out.[4,15,19] In addition, a drain may prevent complete urothelial adhesion to the submucosa. However, temporary low-suction external drainage of this interface has also given good results,[6,7,17] so that no final conclusion can be drawn. Gonzalez *et al.* have suggested continuous intravesical low-pressure maintenance with a bladder catheter to enhance low-pressure distension of the urothelium, with the idea of improving contact of the urothelium with the de-epithelialized patch.[17]

CHOICE OF EXPERIMENTAL MODEL

The well-known ability of a normal bladder to re-expand following partial detrusorectomy has prevented most researchers from producing statistically different data when comparing preoperative and postoperative bladder compliance and capacity.[6,15,25,31] Animal models of neurogenic bladder, i.e., following rhizotomy or an artificial reduction of the capacity of the bladder,[6,35–7] should be used if the long-term urodynamic properties following augmentation cystoplasty are to be evaluated. The 'talc bladder' described by Garibay *et al.* is a small bladder with reduced capacity secondary to a chemically induced intense perivesical inflammatory reaction. It can easily be obtained and appears to retain its poor mechanical properties in the long term.[6] Another way of assessing volume gain following bladder augmentation is by using morphometric analysis of the patches.[14] Although feasible on normal as well as on modified bladders, this technique only assesses the outcome of the size of the patch prior to and following surgery, and does not take into account the mechanical properties of the patches.

The anatomy of the colonic mucosa, submucosa, and muscular layers may differ according to the animal used.

Rats and rabbits have a very thin colonic submucosa, often not detectable macroscopically. Although no technical difficulty has been reported in performing de-epithelialization, intestinal mucosa remnants were often found on the patches, accompanied by secondary inflammation and fibrosis.[8,15,38] These findings are probably related to the difficulty in defining an adequate level for de-epithelialization: too deep and the dissection will injure the muscle, too superficial and the dissection will leave mucosa behind.

The sheep has two thin and delicate colonic muscle layers which may suffer if diathermy dissection is performed.[10]

The minipig has deep colonic mucosa crypts embedded in the submucosa, which render removal of the mucosa tedious at times.[15] Both the sheep and the minipig, as well as the dog and the calf, have a well-defined submucosa which can be injected with normal saline, allowing easier and more adequate de-epithelialization. The minipig has both urinary and terminal intestinal tracts quite similar to those of the human, and may allow reliable long-term histological and urodynamic data assessment. If long-term urodynamics are being assessed, an adequate experimental model of the neurogenic bladder is mandatory, but still to be developed.

EXPERIMENTAL STUDIES

Many studies on various animals have shown that urothelium will grow onto de-epithelialized intestinal segments, by ingrowth from the adjacent bladder wall. This progressive urothelial coverage can take place on both submucosal as well as serosal layers,[8,39] depending on the final orientation of the patch. Some authors have advocated the need for an intact submucosa for adequate urothelial invasion and survival without contraction of the patch.[40] Others have shown that urothelium can invade and survive on various other surfaces such as serosa, peritoneum, omentum, submucosa or gastric muscle stripped of its submucosa.[8,13,14,39,41–3] It seems that the presence of extracellular matrix ligands such as collagen type I, III, and IV, which are found in significant amounts in the submucosa, is important for cell adhesion and growth.[44]

Because of the progressive shrinkage of a de-epithelialized patch in direct contact with urine and because of the poor urodynamic properties of bulging urothelium following autoaugmentation, the merging of both procedures is theoretically very attractive. Some studies have assessed its feasibility on animal models.[4,6,7,9,15,25,26] A follow-up period of more than 1 year is now available with de-epithelialized gastric or colonic segments applied onto an autoaugmentated bladder in the sheep, pig, and dog.[4,6,7,9,11,14,15,25,27] We will first focus on the different studies of experimental autoaugmentation colocystoplasty and then critically review the results.

In the sheep model, Dewan *et al.* compared the postoperative bladder compliance of enterocystoplasties with de-epithelialized sigmoid colon applied on an autoaugmented bladder or on a fully opened bladder. They also assessed intestinal mucosa regrowth on de-epithelialized seromuscular colonic patches following bladder autoaugmentation enterocystoplasties.[26]

In our study using the minipig model, we assessed five techniques of patch coverage of a pedicled, detubularized, and de-epithelialized sigmoid patch. In one group, the patch was applied to intact and protruding urothelium following sagittal detrusoromyotomy. The other groups had either partial or complete urothelial coverage of the patch using various other techniques or else had no urothelial coverage at all.[15]

In the dog model, Garibay *et al.* compared postoperative bladder capacity following detrusorectomy (autoaugmentation) of a normal bladder with that following detrusorectomy of a 'talc bladder' with or without colocystoplasty.[6]

In the dog model, Buson *et al.* compared several seromuscular autoaugmentation techniques using a de-epithelialized colonic patch with or without submucosa, applied on a normal bladder, on a bladder following partial detrusorectomy or applied on a 'talc bladder'.[7]

Denes *et al.* compared the metabolism of ammonium chloride in the normal bladder of dogs following conventional colocystoplasty or seromuscular colocystoplasty with that in an exposed bladder urothelium following subtotal detrusorectomy.[25]

In the dog model, Lima *et al.* proved that autoaugmentation enterocystoplasty with detrusorectomy of normal bladder was feasible and compared it with a group of autoaugmentation alone following detrusoromyotomy.[4]

CONCLUSIONS

The urodynamic data found in each study were based on the results of manometrical studies performed on anesthetized animals with normal bladders, except for two studies on the dog in which 'talc bladders' were used. A significant increase in bladder volume and compliance was obtained only if an autoaugmentation enterocystoplasty was performed on a bladder with an artificially reduced capacity, i.e., 'talc bladder'.

Direct preoperative and postoperative assessments of the mechanical properties of a patch have never been objectively made, although often subjectively described.[9,14,15] It would be interesting to assess more specifically the stress/strain properties of the patch to reliably compare its preoperative and postoperative mechanical properties and outcome. Morphometrical analysis is a reliable way to assess the outcome of the size and shape of the patches,[14] especially when the normal bladder wall does not allow reliable preoperative and postoperative urodynamic data comparison.

Several studies have proved the need for an adequate collagen matrix to be present on the patch in order to enhance urothelial adhesion and survival.[39,45] Furthermore, regular bladder filling and emptying do not seem mandatory for the *in vivo* urothelium islets to survive and grow. Vates *et al.* have shown in a dog model that urothelial islets applied on seromuscular colonic segments covered with silastic and tubularized on a stent could survive and grow to cover the intestinal muscle.[40]

The ideal mechanical properties of the patch to be used for bladder augmentation have not been clearly defined and should be further studied.

Hematoxylin–Eosin and Masson trichrome are the most commonly used staining techniques when assessing the histology of the bladder and its patch.

Intestinal mucosa remnants were described in each study, except in the dog model described by Garibay *et al.* As mentioned previously, on the long-term basis, any intestinal mucosa remnants can theoretically give rise to pathological consequences and should be avoided. However, no common opinion has been reached regarding the most appropriate technique to use. The dilemma concerning the pros and cons of muscularis mucosa removal still remains.[26] On the other hand, the necessity of an adequate coverage of the bulging urothelium to prevent shrinkage has been confirmed.[6]

We have observed, as have others, that a normal urothelial stratification remained on the surface of the patch. The assessment of metabolic acidosis during ammonium chloride loading, as performed by Denes *et al.*, has proved that dogs with autoaugmented colocystoplasties are protected from intravesical ammonium chloride absorption and have normally functioning urothelium. Although this seems to indicate that the surviving urothelium is normal, it remains to be confirmed with a more detailed histological and functional assessment of the surviving urothelium, as well as of the different types of submucosal collagen, using immunohistochemical markers.[45–9]

REFERENCES

1. Cartwright, P.C. and Snow, B.W. (1989) Bladder autoaugmentation; early clinical experience. *Journal of Urology,* **142,** 505–8.
2. Couvelaire, R. (1955) Agrandir la vessie. In Masson eds, *Chirurgie de la Vessie.* Paris, 200–21.
3. Reid, C., Moorhead, J.D. and Hadley, H.R. (1990) Experiences with the detrusorectomy procedure. *Journal of Urology,* **143,** 331A (Abstract 570).
4. Lima, S.V.C., Araujo, L.A.P., Vilar, F.O. *et al.* (1995) Nonsecretory sigmoid cystoplasty: experimental and clinical results. *Journal of Urology,* **153,** 1651–4.
5. Snow, B.W. and Cartwright, M.D. (1991) Bladder augmentation. In King, L.R., Stone, A.R. and Webster, G. (eds.). *Bladder Reconstruction and Continent Urinary Diversion.* Chicargo/London, Year Book Medical: 107–14.
6. Garibay, J.T., Manivel, J.C. and Gonzalez, R. (1995) Effect of seromuscular colocystoplasty lined with urothelium and partial detrusorectomy on a new canine model of reduced bladder capacity. *Journal of Urology,* **154,** 903–6.
7. Buson, H., Manivel, J.C., Dayanc, M. *et al.* (1994) Seromuscular colocystoplasty lined with urothelium: experimental study. *Pediatric Urology,* **44,** 743–8.
8. De Badiola, F., Manivel, J.C. and Gonzalez, R. (1991) Seromuscular enterocystoplasty in rats. *Journal of Urology,* **146,** 559–62.
9. Dewan, P.A., Lorenz, C., Stefanek,W. *et al.* (1994) Urothelial lined colocystoplasty in a sheep model. *European Urology,* **26,** 240–6.
10. Dewan, P.A., Stefanek, W., Lorenz, C. *et al.* (1994) Autoaugmentation omentocystoplasty in the sheep model. *Urology,* **43,** 888–91.
11. Dewan, P.A. and Byard, R.W. (1993) Autoaugmentation gastrocystoplasty in the sheep model. *British Journal of Urology,* **72,** 56–9.
12. Dewan, P.A. and Stefanek, W. (1994) Autoaugmentation colocystoplasty. *Pediatric Surgery International,* **9,** 526–8.
13. Dewan, P.A. Stefanek, W., Lorenz, C. *et al.* (1995) Autoaugmentation gastrocystoplasty and demucosalised gastrocystoplasty in the sheep model. *Urology,* **45,** 291–6.
14. Frey, P., Lutz, N. and Leuba, A.L. (1996) Augmentation cystoplasty using pedicled and de-epithelialised gastric patches in the mini-pig model. *Journal of Urology,* **156,** 608–11.
15. Lutz, N. and Frey, P. (1995) Enterocystoplasty using modified pedicled, detubularised, de-epithelialised sigmoid patches in the mini-pig model. *Journal of Urology,* **154,** 893–8.

16. Gosalbez, R. Jr, Woodard, J.R., Broecker, B.H. *et al.* (1993) The use of stomach in pediatric urinary reconstruction. *Journal of Urology,* **150,** 438–40.
17. Gonzalez, R., Buson, H., Reid, C. *et al.* (1995) Seromuscular colocystoplasty lined with urothelium: experience with 16 patients. *Urology,* **45,** 124–9.
18. Khoury, J.M., Timmons, S.L., Corbel, L. *et al.* (1992) Complications of enterocystoplasty. *Urology,* **40,** 9–14.
19. Campbell, E.W. (1957) Reconstruction of the bladder with a seromuscular graft. *Journal of Urology,* **78,** 236–8.
20. Motley, R.C., Montgomery, B.T., Zollman, P.E. *et al.* (1990) Augmentation cystoplasty utilizing de-epithelialised sigmoid colon: a preliminary study. *Journal of Urology,* **143,** 1257–60.
21. Niku, S.D., Scherz, H.C., Stein, P.C. *et al.* (1995) Intestinal de-epithelialization and augmentation cystoplasty: an animal model. *Urology,* **46,** 36–9.
22. Oesch, I. (1988) Neourothelium in bladder augmentation. An experimental study in rats. *European Urology,* **14,** 328–9.
23. Pippi-Salle, J.L., Fraga, J.C.S., Lucib, A. *et al.* (1990) Seromuscular enterocystoplasty in dogs. *Journal of Urology,* **144,** 454–60.
24. Shoemaker, W.C. (1955) Reversed seromuscular grafts in urinary tract reconstruction. *Journal of Urology,* **74,** 453–75.
25. Denes, E.D., Vates, T.S., Freedman, A.L. *et al.* (1997) Seromuscular colocystoplasty lined with urothelium protects dogs from acidosis during ammonium chloride loading. *Journal of Urology,* **158,** 1075–80.
26. Dewan, P.A., Close, C.E., Byard, R.W. *et al.* (1997) Enteric mucosal regrowth after bladder augmentation using demucosalised gut segments. *Journal of Urology,* **158,** 1141–6.
27. Johnson, H., Nigro, M.K., Stothers, L. *et al.* (1994) Laboratory variables of bladder autoaugmentation in an animal model. *Urology,* **44,** 260–3.
28. Kennelly, M.J., Gormley, A. and McGuire, E.J. (1994) Early clinical experience with adult bladder autoaugmentation. *Journal of Urology,* **152,** 303–6.
29. McDougall, E.M., Clayman, R.V., Figenshau, R.S. *et al.* (1995) Laparoscopic retropubic autoaugmentation of the bladder. *Journal of Urology,* **153,** 123–6.
30. Ehrlich, R.M. and Gershman, A. (1993) Laparoscopic seromyotomy (autoaugmentation) for non-neurogenic neurogenic bladder in a child: initial case report. *Urology,* **42,** 175–8.
31. Figenshau, R.S., Clayman, R.V., Klutke, C.G. *et al.* (1996) Laparoscopic bladder seromyotomy: laboratory experience. *Journal of Endourology,* **10,** 267–71.
32. Gil-Vernet, J.M. Jr (1965) The ileocolic segment in urologic surgery. *Journal of Urology,* **94,** 418–22.
33. Goodwin, W.E., Winter, C.C. and Barker, W.F. (1959) 'Cup patch' technique of ileocystoplasty for bladder enlargement or partial substitution. *Surgery, Gynecology and Obstetrics,* **108,** 240–4.
34. Perito, P.E., Carter, M., Civanto, F. *et al.* Laser-assisted enterocystoplasty in rats. *Journal of Urology,* **150,** 1956–9.
35. O'Brien, D. (1988) Neurogenic disorders of micturition. *Veterinary Clinics of North America – Small Animal Practice,* **18,** 529–44.
36. Vorstman, B., Schlossberg, S., Landy, H. *et al.* (1987) Nerve crossover techniques for urinary bladder reinnervation: animal and human cadaver studies. *Journal of Urology,* **137,** 1043–7.
37. Woodside, J.R., Dail, W.G., McGuire, E.J. *et al.* (1982) The Manx cat as an animal model for neurogenic vesical dysfunction associated with myelodysplasia: a preliminary report. *Journal of Urology,* **127,** 180–3.
38. Merguerian , P., Chavez, D.R. and Hakim, S. (1994) Grafting of cultured uroepithelium and bladder mucosa into de-epithelialised segments of colon in rabbits. *Journal of Urology,* **152,** 671–4.
39. Cheng, E., Rento, R., Grayhack, J.T. *et al.* (1994) Reversed seromuscular flaps in the urinary tract in dogs. *Journal of Urology,* **152,** 2252–7.
40. Vates, T.S., Denes, E.D., Rabah, R. *et al.* (1997) Methods to enhance in vivo urothelial growth on seromuscular colonic segments in the dog. *Journal of Urology,* **158,** 1081–5.
41. Kropp, B.P., Rippy, M.K., Badylak, S.F. *et al.* (1996) Regenerative urinary bladder augmentation using small intestinal submucosa: urodynamic and histopathologic assessment in long-term canine bladder augmentations. *Journal of Urology,* **155,** 2098–104.
42. Weingarten, J.L., Cromie, W.J. and Paty, R.J. (1990) Augmentation myoperitoneocystoplasty. *Journal of Urology,* **144,** 156–8.

43. Goldstein, M.D. and Dearden, L.C. (1966) Histology of omentoplasty of the urinary bladder in the rabbit. *Investigative Urology,* **3,** 460–9.
44. Ludwikowski, B., Zhang, Y.Y. and Frey, P. (1999) The long-term culture of porcine urothelial cells and induction of urothelial stratification. *British Journal of Urology,* **84**, 507–14.
45. Sutherland, R.S., Baskin, L.S., Hayward, S.W. *et al.* (1996) Regeneration of bladder urothelium, smooth muscle, blood vessels and nerves into an acellular tissue matrix. *Journal of Urology,* **156,** 571–7.
46. Cilento, B.G., Freeman, M.R., Scneck, F.X. *et al.* (1994) Phenotypic and cytogenetic characterization of human bladder urothelia expanded in vitro. *Journal of Urology,* **152,** 665–70.
47. Hutton, K.A.R., Trejdosiewicz, L.K., Thomas, D.F.M. *et al.* (1993) Urothelial tissue culture for bladder reconstruction: an experimental study. *Journal of Urology,* **150,** 721–5.
48. Sun, T.T., Zhao, H., Provet, J. *et al.* (1996) Formation of asymmetric unit membrane during urothelial differentiation. *Molecular Biology Reports,* **23,** 3–11.
49. Yu, J., Lin, J.H., Wu, X.R. *et al.* (1994) Uroplakins Ia and Ib, two major differentiation products of bladder epithelium belong to a family of four transmembrane domain (4TM) proteins. *Journal of Cell Biology,* **125,** 171–82.

13

Seromuscular colocystoplasty: clinical experience*

THOMAS S VATES AND RICARDO GONZALEZ

INTRODUCTION

The widespread use of bowel segments has provided many bladder reconstruction options for patients with a small or poorly compliant bladder that is unresponsive to medical therapy. Despite the benefits of bladder augmentation, incorporation of segments of the gastrointestinal tract into the urinary tract can cause undesirable side-effects, specifically: mucus production, chronic bacteruria, stone formation, electrolyte imbalance, perforation, hematuria–dysuria syndrome, and the potential for the development of malignancy.[1–13]

The majority of these adverse effects are due to the absorptive and secretory properties of the gastrointestinal mucosa. When intestinal segments are introduced to the urinary tract, the mechanisms of absorption and secretion remain the same, but the intestinal mucosa is now exposed to new ions, creating a shift in the acid–base balance. It has been well established that absorption of ammonium from urine is the pathophysiological basis of most of the metabolic abnormalities observed in patients who have either large or small bowel interposed in the urinary tract. Ammonium which comes from the metabolism of urea, is reabsorbed with chloride, creating an increased acid load and metabolic acidosis.[4,14–17]

An intriguing option for bladder augmentation which can eliminate several of the undesirable consequences of augmentations based on gastrointestinal segments is the use of urothelial-lined seromuscular intestinal segments. We have studied these augmentations in various animal models and reported the first large series in humans. Since that initial report, we have continued to use this method of bladder augmentation and believe it to be the superior form

*The terms 'autoaugmentation colocystoplasty' and 'seromuscular colocystoplasty' can be used interchangeably and, until international acceptance of nomenclature has been formalized, the authors' preference has been followed.

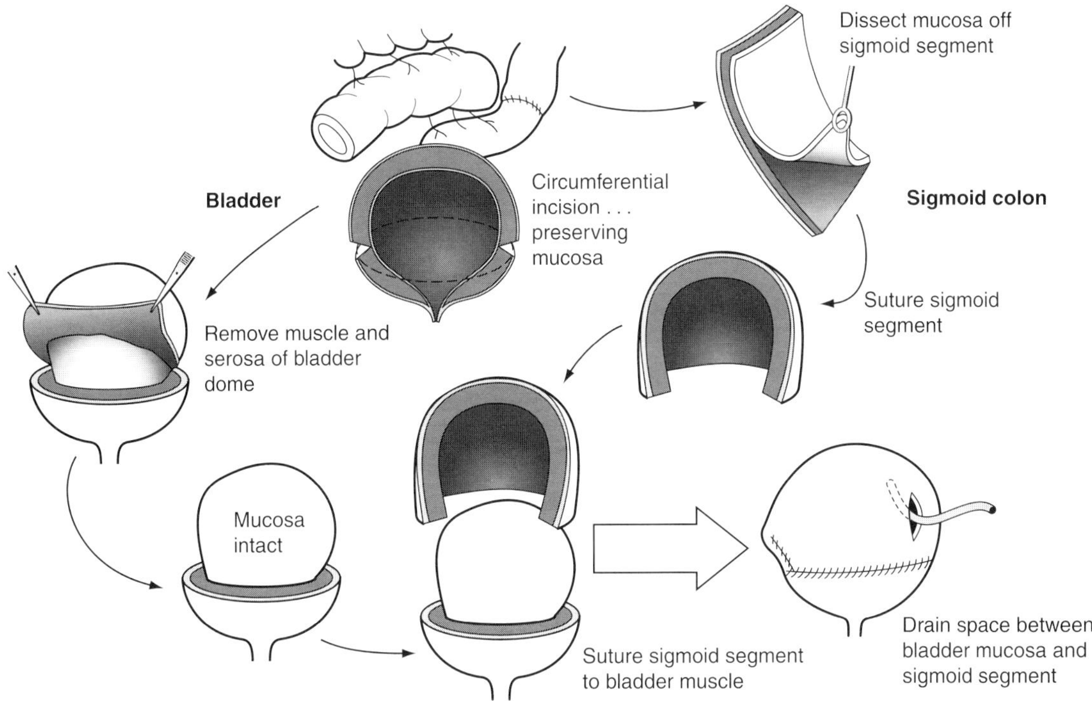

Figure 13.1 *Technique for seromuscular enterocystoplasty lined with urothelium. Reproduced with permission from Figure 1 in Buson, H., Manivel, J.C., Dayanc, M., Long, R. and Gonzalez, R. (1994) Seromuscular colocystoplasty lined with urothelium: experimental study.* Urology, **44** (5), 743–8.

in appropriately selected patients. In this chapter, we review the initial studies on the use of seromuscular intestinal segments for bladder augmentation, and present patient selection criteria and modifications to the operative and postoperative care that have evolved since our initial clinical report on the seromuscular colocystoplasty (SCLU) that we believe enhance its clinical use and success.

The models of seromuscular augmentation can be divided into several categories, but the two most widely and recently studied are: (1) demucosalized gastrointestinal segments anastomosed to the bladder lumen (including reversed and nonreversed seromuscular segments), and (2) demucosalized gastrointestinal segments anastomosed to a bladder which has undergone vesicomyomectomy with preservation of the native urothelium.

CLINICAL STUDIES

Demucosalized bowel anastomosed directly to the bladder lumen

Dewan and Stefanek reported the first case of bladder augmentation using the SCLU technique in a 9-year-old female patient with myelomeningocele. They reported that her bladder capacity increased from 40 cm^3 to 213 cm^3 and she was continent between catheterizations performed every 3 hours.[18] Gonzalez *et al.* reported the first large human experience with the SCLU. The operative procedure involves a detrusomyomectomy (Fig. 13.1), to expose a large portion of intact bladder mucosa, demucosalization of the colonic epithelium, and anastomosing the demucosalized bowel to the bladder over the urothelium. Gonzalez *et al.* describe 16 patients, ten males and six females, with a mean age of 11.7 years. Fourteen patients had neurogenic bladder dysfunction and two had bladder dysfunction secondary to posterior urethral obstruction. Concomitant procedures were performed in 12 patients, including ureteral reimplantation (five), transureteroureterostomy (two), artificial urinary sphincter (one), sigmoid neovagina (one), and cutaneous appendicovesicostomy (one). Postoperative bladder capacity was increased by a mean of 2.4 times and end-filling pressure was decreased by a mean of 50%. Two patients developed an hourglass deformity of the augmented segment, which was easily corrected, and there were two failures who subsequently underwent ileocystoplasty.[19] Lima *et al.* reported the clinical application of the SCLU in ten patients and noted a durable increase in the cystometric capacity of 33–300%.[20] Although Dewan and Stefanek reported the first clinical application of the SCLU, their subsequent clinical studies have focused on the autoaugmentation gastrocystoplasty (AAGC). They described five patients (three males and two females), with a mean age of 12.4 years, with neurogenic bladder dysfunction secondary to myelomeningocele (four) and a cerebrovascular accident (one) who underwent AAGC. Four patients underwent urodynamic evaluation at 3 and 12 months post operatively, with improvement in bladder capacity and bladder compliance. However, one patient required a revision 3 months post operatively; two patients still had episodes of incontinence; and three had transient intolerance of large meals.[21] Although the stomach may be the organ of choice for some, we feel the colon, a nonvital organ which is in anatomic proximity to the bladder and thus easier to use, is superior to the stomach. The only advantages offered by the stomach are its secretory properties, which are eliminated when the mucosa is removed.

Since our initial report of the clinical experience with SCLU, we have utilized this technique in another 13 patients, eight females and five males, with a mean age of 7.8 years. All patients had neurogenic bladder dysfunction secondary to myelodysplasia. Of the 13 patients, nine were successfully augmented, three were failures, and one was lost to follow-up. In the successful group, the mean safe bladder capacity increased from 139 cm^3 to 305 cm^3 ($p<0.001$) and the mean end cystometric filling pressure decreased from 71 cmH_2O to 28 cmH_2O ($p<0.005$). However, there were also three failures (two females and one male). In all patients who failed, the bladder was not distended in the early postoperative period. Neither of the females had a bladder neck procedure and one had a ureteral reimplant with urinary extravasation. The male patient did have an artificial urinary sphincter placed at the same time as the SCLU, but this was not activated early.[22] In addition, all patients who had an artificial urinary sphincter placed prior to the SCLU were successfully augmented. This series suggests that SCLU failures are associated with inability to maintain adequate bladder distension in the early postoperative period, due either to failure to increase bladder outlet resistance or concomitant bladder procedures.

Based on this series we believe the ideal candidate for SCLU should have intact urothelium and a bladder neck procedure (sling, cinch, or artificial sphincter) to maintain bladder distension. Patients having concomitant bladder surgery which violates the integrity of the urothelium or could result in urinary extravasation (i.e., ureteral reimplantation or appendicovesicostomy) and patients with severely trabeculated bladders in whom performing the vesicomyomectomy will result in multiple holes in the urothelium should not have an SCLU. If an SCLU is contemplated in a patient with vesicoureteral reflux, we recommend a staged procedure with the antireflux surgery being performed first.

The only modification to the operative procedure since the initial series has been the abandonment of the use of a Penrose drain between the native urothelium and seromuscular colonic segment. As stated earlier, we feel early bladder distension is crucial to enable the intact urothelium to adhere to the demucosalized colonic segment and thus result in a successful augmentation. To achieve this, we use a urinary drainage catheter with a vent placed 30 cm above the patient's pubis. We do not use a suprapubic tube as this might impair mucosal adherence to the seromuscular segment and these patients do not produce visible mucus.

POSTOPERATIVE CARE

Postoperative care is straightforward for most patients. As we use colon for our seromuscular segment, we routinely remove the nasogastric tube on the second postoperative day. Oral intake is based on return of gastrointestinal function and varies considerably for each patient. The urinary drainage is not usually grossly blood stained: if blood staining does occur, a mucosal injury should be suspected and consideration given to prolonged urethral drainage. Routinely, the urethral catheter is removed on the fourth postoperative day, and patients start clean intermittent catheterization. A small amount of hematuria with the first or second catheterization is not a cause for concern, but if blood persists or catheterization is difficult, or if the patient is leaking between catheterizations, then one should again be concerned that mucosal adherence to the seromuscular segment may be compromized. We employ the same postoperative imaging and electrolyte studies for children with SCLU as we do for conventional augmentation cystoplasties.

CONCLUSIONS

In conclusion, we believe the SCLU is a viable option for bladder augmentation in the appropriate patient. It is particularly well suited to the child who is at greatest risk for metabolic abnormalities, which may affect growth. Bladder distension early in the postoperative period is crucial to allow the urothelium to adhere to the seromuscular segment, and procedures that violate the native urothelium should not be performed concomitantly with a SCLU. Although clinical experience with the SCLU is still limited, it appears to be a method of bladder augmentation with merit and deserving further clinical investigation.

REFERENCES

1. Gonzalez, R. (1993) Bladder augmentation with sigmoid colon. In Webster, G., King, L. and Goldwasser, B. (eds.). *Reconstructive Urology.* Blackwell Scientific, Oxford: 433–8.
2. Mitchell, M.E. and Burns, M. (1993) Autoaugmentation cystoplasty with stomach. In Webster, G., King, L. and Goldwasser, B. (eds.). *Reconstructive Urology.* Blackwell Scientific, Oxford: 439–44.
3. Nurse, D.E. and Mundy, A.R. (1989) Metabolic complications of cystoplasty. *British Journal of Urology,* **63,** 165–70.
4. McDougal, W.S. (1992) Metabolic complications of urinary intestinal diversion. *Journal of Urology,* **147,** 1199.
5. Blyth, B., Ewalt, D.H., Duckett, J.W. *et al.* (1992) Lithogenic properties of enterocystoplasty. *Journal of Urology,* **148 (Part 2),** 575–7.
6. Palmer, L.S., Franco, I., Kogan, S.J. *et al.* (1993) Urolithiasis in children following augmentation cystoplasty. *Journal of Urology,* **150,** 726–8.
7. Bauer, S.B., Hendren, W.H., Kozakewich, H. *et al.* (1992) Perforation of the augmented bladder. *Journal of Urology,* **148** (Part 2), 669–703.
8. Filmer, R.B. and Spencer, J.R. (1990) Malignancies in bladder augmentation and intestinal conduits. *Journal of Urology,* **143,** 671–8.
9. Treiger, B.F.G. and Marshall, F.F. (1991) Carcinogenesis and the use of intestinal segments in the urinary tract. *Urologic Clinics of North America,* **18,** 737.
10. Buson, H., Castro-Diaz, D., Manivel, J.C. *et al.* (1993) The development of tumors in experimental gastrocystoplasty. *Journal of Urology,* **150,** 730–3.
11. Nguyen, D.H., Bain, M.A., Salmonson, K.L. *et al.* (1993) The syndrome of dysuria–hematuria in npediatric urinary reconstruction with stomach. *Journal of Urology,* **150,** 707–9.
12. Plawker, M.W., Rabinowitz, S.S., Etwaru, D.J. *et al.* (1995) Hypergastrinemia, dysuria, hematuria and metabolic alkalosis: complications associated with gastrocystoplasty. *Journal of Urology,* **154,** 546–9.
13. Reinberg, Y., Manivel, J., Froemming, C. *et al.* (1992) Perforation of the gastric segment of an augmented bladder secondary to peptic ulcer disease. *Journal of Urology,* **148,** 369–71.
14. Hall, M.C., Koch, M.O. and McDougal, W.S. (1991) Metabolic consequences of urinary diversion through intestinal segments. *Urologic Clinics of North America,* **18,** 725.

15. Koch, M.O., McDougal, W.S., Reddy, P.K. *et al.* (1991) Metabolic alterations following continent urinary diversion through colonic segments. *Journal of Urology,* **145,** 270.
16. Koch, M.O., Gurevitch, E., Hill, D.E. *et al.* (1990) Urinary solute transport by intestinal segments: a comparative study of ileum and colon in rats. *Journal of Urology,* **143,** 1275–9.
17. Koch, M.O. and McDougal, W.S. (1985) The pathophysiology of hyperchloremic metabolic acidosis after urinary diversion through intestinal segments. *Surgery,* **98,** 561.
18. Dewan, P.A. and Stefanek, W. (1994) Autoaugmentation colocystoplasty. *Pediatric Surgery International,* **9,** 526–8.
19. Gonzalez, R., Buson, H., Reid, C. *et al.* (1995) Seromuscular colocystoplasty lined with urothelium: experience with 16 patients. *Urology,* **45**, 124–9.
20. Lima, S.V.C., Araujo, L.A.P., Vilar, F.O. *et al.* (1995) Non-secretory sigmoid cystoplasty: experimental and clinical results. *Journal of Urology,* **153,** 1651–4.
21. Dewan, P.A. and Stefanek, W. (1994) Autoaugmentation gastrocystoplasty: early clinical results. *British Journal of Urology,* **74,** 460–4.
22. Vates, T.S., Smith, C.A. and Gonzalez, R.G. (1997) Importance of early bladder distension for the success of the seromuscular colocystoplasty lined with urothelium (SCLU). American Academy of Pediatrics Annual Meeting, November.

14

Bladder regeneration technology

BRADLEY P KROPP AND RICHARD C RINK

INTRODUCTION

Over the past two decades there have been tremendous advances in lower urinary tract reconstruction. We are now at the point where we can reliably reconstruct the entire urinary tract and provide continence. These major reconstructions have primarily used a segment of the gastrointestinal tract. While this has dramatically improved the lifestyle of many patients with severe neurogenic or anatomic abnormalities, it has also resulted in a new set of risks and complications, including infection, intestinal obstruction, electrolyte abnormalities, metabolic disturbances, bladder perforation, and the potential for tumor production. Recent interest in bladder regeneration technology has been cultivated due to these possible side-effects. Therefore, a material that is readily available, will increase bladder volume and compliance, does not violate the gastrointestinal tract, is nonimmunogenic, and will promote bladder regeneration would be a great addition to the armamentarium of the genitourinary reconstructive surgeon.

HISTORICAL BACKGROUND

The concept of bladder regeneration is not a new phenomenon and has been well documented in the literature over the past century.[1] The major obstacle has been finding a biomaterial, either permanent or biodegradable, that will act as a suitable scaffold for this natural process to occur. Attempts with permanent biomaterials began in 1955, when Bohne *et al.* demonstrated that bladder regeneration will occur in dogs over an acrylic mold.[2] Mortality and complication rates were high, secondary to ureteral strictures, pyelonephritis and peritonitis. However, two dogs did survive for more than 6 months and were histologically shown to have bladder regeneration. Kudish, in 1957, reported poor results using a permanent polyvinyl sponge as a patch for bladder replacement in dogs.[3] Sponges fail to incorporate with the normal bladder tissue and all the implants were partially extruded into the bladder lumina. In 1957, Bohne and Urwiller reported on the first humans in whom a permanent polyethylene mold was used to promote bladder regeneration.

Complications in this series included urinary tract infections, hydronephrosis, fistula formation, and contraction of the regenerated bladder. Despite the poor clinical results, he was able to prove that bladder regeneration will occur in human bladders given the proper scaffold.[4] In 1961, Swinney *et al.*, using Teflon for partial bladder replacement, were able to demonstrate uroepithelium regeneration, but not smooth muscle regeneration.[5] They also experienced graft extrusion and a fibrous bladder regeneration which led to the ultimate failure of this material.

Tsuji *et al.* did most of the experimental and clinical work associated with the gelatin sponge.[6] In 1967, they reported their work with 23 rabbits that underwent partial bladder replacement with a gelatin sponge which had been emersed in 99% ethyl alcohol. Eight animals died as a consequence of urinary extravasation, with the remaining 15 rabbits showing both mucosal and detrusor muscle regeneration at 4 months. That same year, Tsuji *et al.* also reported on the use of the gelatin sponge in humans; however, their patients suffered poor results due to 'neobladder' contraction and hydronephrosis.[7] In 1970, Orikasa and Tsuji reported excellent results in four of five cystoplasties in humans where gelatin sponges were sprayed with nobecutane.[8] Their one failure was in a patient with a severely contracted bladder, who suffered an early postoperative leak due to a malfunctioning catheter. Bladder biopsy in one patient 8 months postoperatively showed excellent mucosal and muscle regeneration. Unfortunately, long-term follow-up of these patients has not been reported.

Attempts have also been made to use Silastic patches for partial bladder replacement; however, these, too, have been complicated by persistent infections, graft extrusion, and stone formation. In one series, only one dog that did not develop an infection had successful muscle regeneration.[9] Stanley *et al.* reported using silicone rubber bladder prostheses covered with Dacron velour to prevent exposure of the rubber. They reported good results at 1 year in both sheep and dogs. Mucosal and muscle regeneration did occur, but at a much slower rate than in previously reported cases.[10]

In addition to the above permanent materials, attempts have been made to find a biodegradable material that would function as a scaffold and also allow for bladder regeneration. Taguchi *et al.* reported the use of thin Japanese paper treated with nobecutane,[11] while Scott *et al.* have reported good regenerative capacity with collagen/Vicryl composite membrane implants used for renal capsules, ureteral wall, and bladder wall replacement.[12] Kelami used lyophilized human dura and obtained good functional results, both experimentally and clinically. However, evidence of smooth muscle fibers was seen in only one case.[13] The use of this material is also limited due to its expense, propensity for contraction, metaplastic bone formation, and incomplete reabsorption. In 1987, Fishman and associates were able to show that amniotic tissue was an excellent, inexpensive, biodegradable, hypoallergenic graft material that could have potential use in the reconstruction of the urinary tract of dogs.[14] Finally, in 1992, Kambic *et al.* reported on the use of biodegradable pericardial implants for bladder augmentation in dogs. Functionally, these implanted bladders demonstrated adequate bladder capacity for up to 36 months, but grossly they were noted to have graft shrinkage. Histologically, there was a smooth epithelialized inner surface but absence of a smooth muscle layer.[15] Therefore, although pericardial tissue can be used to replace part of the bladder wall, it does not appear to promote complete bladder regeneration, which appears to be important for eventual long-term compliance and success.

CURRENT TECHNOLOGY

Despite the urinary bladder's natural ability to repair and remodel itself, urologists have been unable to find a suitable scaffold material to give consistent and reliable regenerative results. Currently, two technologies for bladder regeneration and augmentation are being investigated.

The first technology involves tissue engineering techniques using biodegradable materials which act as cell-delivery vehicles. In 1992, Atala *et al.* demonstrated the successful use of a nonwoven polyglycolic acid polymer to allow the *in vitro* growth of rabbit and human bladder epithelium and smooth muscle cells.[16] Remarkably, they were further able to demonstrate that human urothelium and smooth muscle cells grown on the biodegradable polymers could then be implanted into athymic mice and grown *in vivo* with further expansion of the epithelium and smooth muscle layers. Cilento *et al.* demonstrated that by using this method of cell culture, it would be theoretically possible to expand a urothelial strain to cover the area of an entire football field.[17] Recently, Yoo *et al.* reported the feasibility of bladder augmentation using biodegradable polymer scaffolds seeded with urothelial and smooth muscle cells.[18] The study showed urothelial and smooth muscle cells could be harvested and expanded separately and the cells could then be seeded on to sheets of polyglycolic acid polymers *in vitro*. The polymer–cell complexes were then used for bladder augmentations in dogs. Urodynamic studies between 6 and 12 weeks demonstrated a 40% and 30% increase in bladder capacity and compliance, respectively. Histologically, the implants of the polymer–cell complexes were all noted to contain a normal cellular organization consisting of uroepithelium and smooth muscle ingrowth. Interestingly, the polymers without cell complexes were also shown to have evidence of bladder regeneration. Therefore, it is yet to be determined whether the sophisticated tissue engineering techniques and monumental contributions that Dr Atala has made to advance the fields of cell culture and tissue engineering will be necessary in the urinary bladder, which so readily regenerates itself.

The second technology for bladder regeneration currently being investigated is the development of biodegradable, acellular, autologous or xenogenic, collagen-based tissue matrix grafts, derived from stomach, bladder, and small intestine. These collagen-based acellular matrix grafts function as a temporary scaffold to promote and allow for the bladder to naturally regenerate.

Sutherland *et al.* reported bladder regeneration in the rat using a free graft of acellular tissue matrix.[19] The tissue matrix was obtained as an allograft from rat stomach or bladder, treated with distilled water, sodium deoxycholate and deoxyribosenuclease. A partial cystectomy (compromising 25% of the bladder) was performed in a rat model and the graft material was then used for augmentation cystoplasty. They demonstrated that the urothelium completely covered the matrix by 4 days and neovascularity was detected at 7 days. Smooth muscle was also detected in the matrix at 14 days, and by 30 days had completely traversed the matrix. They postulated that the regenerated epithelium was inducing the development of smooth muscle. Nerve fiber ingrowth into the acellular matrix was noted by 4 weeks. Findings for both bladder and gastric acellular matrices were similar. This study further supports the rapid rate at which the bladder will regenerate, but, most importantly, suggests that cell–cell signaling occurs between the epithelium and the mesenchyme, via the extracellular matrix, to facilitate the induction and development of bladder smooth muscle and bladder regeneration.

Another collagen-based biomaterial which has recently emerged is the small intestinal submucosal (SIS) graft.[20] This is a xenogenic membrane harvested from pig small intestine, in which the tunica muscularis are mechanically removed from the outer surface. This produces a thin, translucent graft (0.1 mm wall thickness) composed mainly of the submucosal layer of the bowel wall, but which does have the stratum compactum and muscularis mucosa of the tunica mucosa attached. Production of SIS is similar to the manufacturing of sausage casing. Additionally, the submucosal layer of animal intestine has long been used in surgery as gut suture. This collagen-rich membrane has been previously shown to function well as an arterial or venous graft, with rapid replacement by native tissues.[20–2] It was also shown to have excellent host compatibility and remodeling when submucosal bladder injection of minced SIS was performed in pigs.[23] To date, SIS has been shown to be nonimmunogenic, with over 1000 cross-species transplants and direct challenge testing elucidating no response.[24,25]

The initial research done with SIS for urinary bladder augmentations was performed in the rat model. It was shown that SIS functioned as a scaffold to allow the native rat bladder to remodel and regenerate itself. Histologically, the regenerated rat bladders contained all three layers of the bladder (urothelium, smooth muscle, and serosa) and were indistinguishable from normal rat bladder at 11 months postaugmentation.[26] Vaught *et al.* demonstrated through *in vitro* contractility studies that strips of SIS-regenerated rat bladder had contractile properties and innervation similar to control animals.[27] In addition to supporting the regenerative potential of detrusor smooth muscle and nerves, these studies demonstrated that the rat was a poor augmentation model and that further research must be performed in a long-term, large animal model.

Recently, Kropp *et al.* demonstrated that in a canine SIS-augmentation model, in which 40% of the bladder was removed and replaced with a similar-sized piece of SIS, the bladder remained urodynamically compliant, with similar capacities to those of control dogs, while causing no deleterious side-effects or upper tract changes up to 15 months postaugmentation. Histologically, all three layers of the bladder had regenerated. However, the quantity and organization of smooth muscle fibers differed slightly from the normal bladder.[28] In addition, *in vitro* contractility bladder strip studies, on only the SIS-generated portions of the bladder, demonstrated contractile activity and expression of muscarinic, adrenergic, and purinergic receptors similar to those of normal bladder. Furthermore, SIS-regenerated bladder also demonstrated functional nerve regeneration and innervation that are similar to those of normal bladder. Finally, *in vitro* stress/strain compliance studies demonstrated no significant difference between SIS-regenerated bladder and control bladder, both of which were 30–fold more compliant than the original SIS graft material.[29]

The above work with SIS-regenerated bladder augmentations in a large animal model supports the theory that native normal bladder will regenerate itself without complications, thereby having some potential clinical ramifications. However, the ultimate clinical question that remains is: how will an abnormal bladder respond to the presently unknown stimuli that SIS possess?

In order to better define the stimuli that SIS contains, Pope *et al.* used the SIS material to define the early regenerative events that occur in the canine bladder. They demonstrated prominent neovascularization throughout the entire graft very early after implantation. Epithelialization of the graft surface was complete by 3 weeks and demonstrated normal transitional histology. Smooth muscle formation appeared to begin at 2 weeks from dense parallel sheets of elongated smooth muscle actin-positive spindle cells emanating from the incized native smooth muscle margins and running parallel to the mucosal surface. This spindle cell proliferation completely traverses the graft by 4 weeks. These spindle-shaped cells differentiated into smooth muscle bundles by 8 to 10 weeks. Pope *et al.* were also able to demonstrate that nerve ingrowth appeared to coincide with the ingrowth of muscle-forming spindle cells.[30]

The above research demonstrated that SIS was serving as a scaffold for the native bladder to regenerate itself. However, it is known that SIS contains a combination of cytokines, structural proteins, growth factors, glycoproteins, and proteoglycans that may assist in the cell migration, cell to extracellular matrix interaction, and cell growth and differentiation during the regenerative process.[31] To better assess the potential contributions of these factors, Cheng has preliminary evidence that both SIS sheets and SIS gel (partial digest of SIS) support human stroma cell growth. The growth pattern on both forms of SIS demonstrates organized cells in multiple layers with matrix penetrance. From this research, it is tempting to speculate that the SIS material is providing both a scaffold and naturally occurring growth factors to improve the regenerative capacity of the bladder.[32]

CONCLUSIONS

The above technologies being investigated have proven conclusively that the bladder has the ability to regenerate itself, given the proper scaffold. It would appear that a biodegradable material covered with urothelial and smooth muscle cells, from either an *in vitro*[16] or an *in vivo*[19,28] process, is the most clinically plausible. Current technologies in bladder regeneration could provide for the development of a material that could replace the use of bowel for urinary reconstruction in the future. In addition, the current research is greatly expanding the knowledge of bladder development, growth factors, and signals responsible for bladder regeneration.

REFERENCES

1. Tizzoni, G. and Poggi, A. (1888) Die Wiederherstellung der Harnblase: experimentelle

Untersuchungen. *Zentralblatt für Chirurgie,* **15,** 921–6.

2. Bohne, A.W., Osborn, R.W. and Hettle, P.J. (1955) Regeneration of the urinary bladder in the dog, following total cystectomy. *Surgery, Gynaecology and Obstetrics,* **100,** 259–68.
3. Kudish, H.G. (1957) The use of polyvinyl sponge for experimental cystoplasty. *Journal of Urology,* **78,** 232–40.
4. Bohne, A.W. and Urwiller, K.L. (1957) Experience with urinary bladder regeneration. *Journal of Urology,* **77,** 725–32.
5. Swinney, J., Tomlinson, B.E. and Walder, D.N. (1961) Urinary tract substitution. *British Journal of Urology,* **33,** 414.
6. Tsuji, I., Shiraishi, Y., Kassai, T. *et al.* (1967) Further experimental investigations on bladder reconstruction without using the intestine. *Journal of Urology,* **97,** 1021–8.
7. Tsuji, I., Kuroda, K., Fujieda, J. *et al.* (1967) Clinical experiences of bladder reconstruction using preserved bladder and gelatin sponge bladder in the case of bladder cancer. *Journal of Urology,* **98,** 91–2.
8. Orikasa, S. and Tsuji, I. (1970) Enlargement of contracted bladder by use of gelatin sponge bladder. *Journal of Urology,* **104,** 107–10.
9. Ashkar, L.N. and Davis, W.G. (1969) Silastic repair of ureteropelvic junction stricture. *Journal of Urology,* **101,** 801–2.
10. Stanley, T.H., Feminella, J.J., Priestley, J.B. *et al.* (1972) Subtotal cystectomy and prosthetic bladder replacement. *Journal of Urology,* **107,** 783–7.
11. Taguchi, H., Ishizuka, E. and Saito, K. (1977) Cystoplasty by regeneration of the bladder. *Journal of Urology,* **118,** 752–6.
12. Scott, R., Mohammed, R., Gorham, S.D. *et al.* (1988) The evolution of a biodegradable membrane for use in urological surgery. A summary of 109 *in vivo* experiments. *British Journal of Urology,* **62,** 26–31.
13. Kelami, A. (1971) Lyophilized human dura as a bladder wall substitute: experimental and clinical results. *Journal of Urology,* **105,** 518–22.
14. Fishman, I.J., Flores, F.N., Scott, B. *et al.* (1987) Use of fresh placental membranes for bladder reconstruction. *Journal of Urology,* **138,** 1291.
15. Kambic, H., Kay, R., Chen, J.F. *et al.* (1992) Biodegradable pericardial implants for bladder augmentation: a 2.5 year study in dogs. *Journal of Urology,* **147** 539–43.
16. Atala, A., Vacanti, J.P., Peters, C.A. *et al.* (1992) Formation of urothelial structures *in vivo* from dissociated cells attached to biodegradable polymer scaffolds *in vitro*. *Journal of Urology,* **148,** 658–62.
17. Cilento, B.G., Freeman, M.R., Schneck, F.X. *et al.* (1994) Phenotypic and cytogenetic characterization of human bladder urothelia expanded *in vitro*. *Journal of Urology,* **152,** 665–70.
18. Yoo, J.J., Satar, N. and Atala, A. (1995) Bladder augmentation using biodegradable polymer scaffolds seeded with urothelial and smooth muscle cells. Presented at American Academy of Pediatrics, Urology Section, San Francisco.
19. Sutherland, R.S., Baskin, L.S., Hayward, S.W. *et al.* (1996) Regeneration of bladder urothelium, smooth muscle, blood vessels and nerves into an acellular tissue matrix. *Journal of Urology,* **156,** 571.
20. Badylak, S.F., Lantz, G.C., Coffey, A. *et al.* (1989) Small intestinal submucosa as a large diameter vascular graft in the dog. *Journal of Surgical Research,* **47,** 74–80.
21. Lantz, G.C., Badylak, S.F., Coffey, A.C. *et al.* (1990) Small intestinal submucosa as a small diameter arterial graft in the dog. *Journal of Investigative Surgery,* **3,** 217–27.
22. Lantz, G.C., Badylak, S.F., Coffey, A.C. *et al.* (1992) Small intestinal submucosa as a superior vena cava graft in the dog. *Journal of Surgical Research,* **53,** 175.
23. Knapp, P.M., Lingeman, J.E. andSiegal, Y.I. (1994) Biocompatibility of small intestinal submucosa in urinary tract as augmentation cystoplasty graft and injectable suspension. *Journal of Endourology,* **8,** 125–30.
24. Badylak, S.F. (1994) The immunogenic response of SIS. Personal communication.
25. *Metzger, D.W., Moyad, T.F., McPherson, T.* et al. *(1996) Cytokine and antibody responses to xenogeneic SIS transplants. Presented at the First SIS Symposium, Orlando, Florida, December 11.*
26. *Kropp, B.P., Eppley, B.L., Prevel, C.D.* et al. (1995) Experimental assessment of small intestine submucosa as a bladder wall substitute. *Urology,* **46,** 396–400.

27. Vaught, J.D., Kropp, B.P., Sawyer, B.D. *et al.* (1996) Detrusor smooth muscle regeneration in the rat using porcine small intestinal submucosal grafts: functional innervation and receptor expression. *Journal of Urology,* **155,** 374–8.
28. Kropp, B.P., Rippy, M.K., Badylak, S.F. *et al.* (1996) Regenerative urinary bladder augmentation using small intestinal submucosa: urodynamic and histopathologic assessment in long-term canine bladder augmentations. *Journal of Urology,* **155,** 2098–104.
29. Kropp, B.P., Sawyer, B.D., Shannon, H.E. *et al.* (1996) Characterization of small intestinal submucosa regenerated canine detrusor: assessment of reinnervation, *in vitro* compliance and contractility. *Journal of Urology,* **156,** 599–607.
30. Pope, J.C. IV, Davis, M.M., Smith, E.R. Jr *et al.* (1997) The ontogeny of canine SIS-regenerated urinary bladder. *Journal of Urology,* **158**(3 Pt 2), 1105–10.
31. Badylak, S.F. (1996) Speculation (with a little evidence) for the roles of cell proliferation, differentiation, neovascularization, and environmental stressors in SIS induced remodeling. Presented at the First SIS Symposium, Orlando, Florida, December 11.
32. Cheng, E. (1997) Cell culture with SIS. Personal communication.

15

The scientific basis of bladder augmentation*

LAURENCE S BASKIN AND GERALD CUNHA

INTRODUCTION

The urinary bladder has two major functions: (a) storage; and (b) socially acceptable, efficient emptying.[1] In children born with neurogenic bladders, coordinated voiding is rarely possible.[2] Starting from the newborn period, these patients can achieve effective bladder emptying with intermittent catheterization.[3] The major issue confronting this group of patients is urinary storage. To accomplish this task, extensive efforts have gone into creating compliant reservoirs.[4] These low-pressure, adequate volume reservoirs must have sufficient outlet resistance to assure urinary continence. Initial treatment involves pharmacologic manipulation, typically with anticholinergic medication.[2] When this proves inadequate, bladder augmentation is the next step. The goal of this chapter is to review the basic science of bladder augmentation.

PRESENT AUGMENTATION STRATEGIES

For the bladder to be a safe and effective storage chamber, the ideal cellular lining is urothelium. Epithelial cells from the gastrointestinal tract are not optimal for this purpose because they either secrete or absorb electrolytes.[5,6] This can lead to chronic electrolyte abnormalities, such as metabolic acidosis, as occurs with ileal augmentation cystoplasties. In the case of gastric augmentations, the stomach segment continues to act as a gastric secreting organ which may predispose to hypochloremic hypokalemic metabolic alkalosis.[7,8] Chronic electrolyte imbalance may also lead to abnormalities in calcium homeostasis, resulting in bone demineralization. The risk of tumors in bladder augmentation seems to be increased, based on sporadic case reports and experimental studies.[9,10] Intestinal segments also secrete mucus, changing the quality of urine in these patients. The use of bowel in the urinary tract also increases the chance of urolithiasis through unknown lithogenic properties.[11]

A number of strategies have been devized to avoid the use of bowel in the urinary tract. Autoaugmentation, as described by Cartwright and Snow, has had success in a select group of patients whose compliance is poor based on abnormal pressures.[12] This procedure is technically difficult in patients who have poor volumes secondary to small contracted bladders. The concept of creating a large bladder

*Supported by NIH Grants K08 DK02397-04, R01 DK51397-02 and DK57246-01.

diverticulum composed of urothelium and lamina propria has been extended by attempting to support the inherently weak autoaugment with de-epithelialized bowel segments from the stomach or the sigmoid colon.[13,14] The well-vascularized, de-epithelialized bowel segments can theoretically provide a vascularized stromal support to the urothelial diverticulum. What type of cellular interactions occur at this foreign interface between bladder urothelial cells and intestinal stroma? Before we can answer this question, we first need to define what we mean by 'normal' urothelium, stroma, and extracellular matrix.

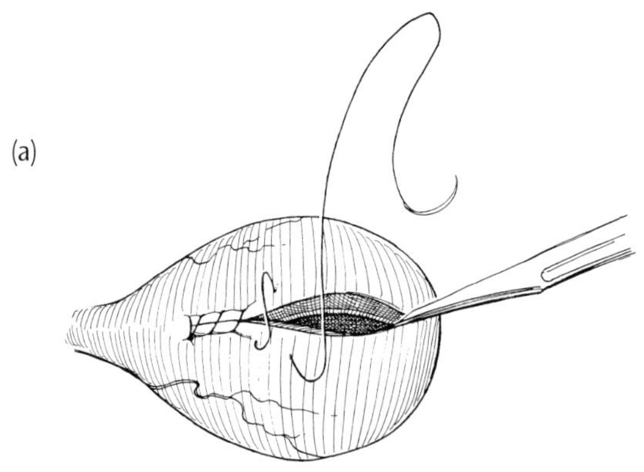

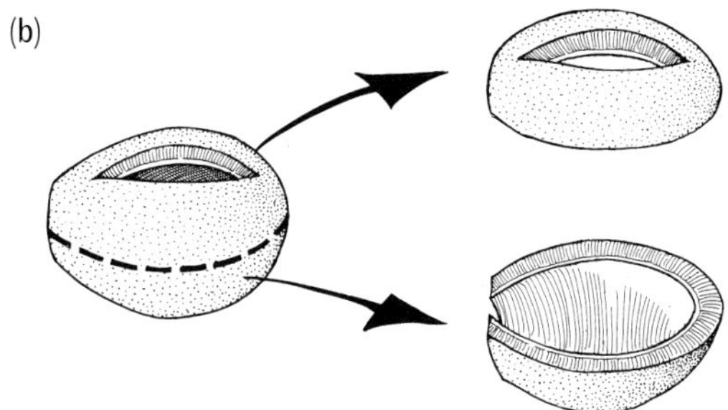

Figure 15.1 *Diagram of bladder wound healing model. (a) Surgical incision. (b) Harvesting and processing technique anterior bladder half = wounded; posterior bladder half = nonwounded. Reproduced with permission from Baskin, L.* et al *(1997) Growth factors in bladder wound healing.* Journal of Urology, ***157****, 2388–95.*

DEFINING UROTHELIUM

As previously stated, the ideal goal of bladder augmentation is to have a urothelial cell-lined bladder. To accomplish this goal we need to carefully define the phenotype of the urothelial cell. Currently, urothelium can be defined by morphology, protein expression, turnover, and function. Histologically, bladder urothelium is a stratified transitional epithelium consisting of basal, intermediate, and superficial cells. Functionally, these cells must accommodate rapid changes in volume and pressure.[15] During bladder cycling, the urothelial cells function as an impermeable barrier to most solutes. The superficial urothelial cells have a highly specialized apical membrane consisting of thickened plaques of asymmetric unit membrane which can be internalized to decrease the luminal surface area of the bladder during emptying. The asymmetric unit membrane is composed of urothelial-specific proteins, the uroplakins.[16]

It is possible to culture urothelial cells *in vitro*[17–22] Depending on the *in vitro* environment, the urothelial cells can form a monolayer or can be induced to stratify and mimic the *in vivo* phenotype. Southgate *et al.* have been able to show that long-term organ cultures of urothelium retain the same basic phenotype as normal urinary tract tissue *in situ*. The 'normal' phenotype is based on the addition of the exogenous calcium to the *in vitro* cultures, as well as the presence of the proper stroma.[21]

It is therefore possible to develop a table of antigen expression for urothelium *in situ* and compare the phenotype to urothelium during cell culture, and to urothelium that has been placed in the environment of a different stroma, such as is occurring in bladder reconstruction (Table 15.1). The antigen expression of cytokeratins, uroplakins, integrins, and E-cadherin has been well described.[16,18,23] As we learn more about urothelial cells, and as new markers become available, we will be able to expand on the antigen expression. These data will be useful, both experimentally and clinically, in defining normal urothelium.

Urothelium can also be defined based on metabolic rate. In the natural state, urothelial cells have an extremely low mitotic activity, remaining quiescent until the need arises for proliferation.[24] In fact,

Table 15.1 *Immunofluorescence on normal human urothelial tissue sections, cultured urothelial cells, and intact organ cultures*

Antibody	Type/specificity*	Normal urothelial tissue			Cultured urothelial cells	Intact organ culture		
		Basal	Inter-mediate	Super-ficial		Basal	Inter-mediate	Super-ficial
LdS68	Monoclonal keratin 7	++	++	++	++			
LdS103	Monoclonal keratin 7,8,18	++	++	++	++			
LP1K	Monoclonal keratin 7	++	++	++	++			
E3	Monoclonal keratin 17	++	++	++	++/+			
BA16	Monoclonal keratin 19	++	++	++	++			
LP2K	Monoclonal keratin 19	++	++	++	+++/+	++	++	+++
LE41	Monoclonal keratin 8	+	+	++	+	+	+	++
LE61	Monoclonal keratin 18	+	+	++	++	+	+	++
CAM5.2	Monoclonal keratin 18,19	+	+	++	+++/++			
2D7	Monoclonal keratin 13†	++	++	–	++			
IC7	Monoclonal keratin 13†	++	++	–	++			
KS13.1	Monoclonal keratin 13	++	++	–	++			
CK8.6	Monoclonal keratin 1,10,11	–	–	–	–			
KB37	Monoclonal basal, squamous	–	–	–	–			
6B10	Monoclonal keratin 4	–	–	–	–			
LL001	Monoclonal keratin 14	–	–	–	++			
AUM	Rabbit urothelial membrane antigen	+	+	+++	–	+	+	+/–
ASU	Rabbit asymmetric unit membrane	–	–	++	–			
AE31	Monoclonal uroplakin 1	–	–	++	–			
V9	Monoclonal vimentin	–	–	–	++			
L9	Rabbit fibronectin	–	–	–	++			
F4	Monoclonal fibronectin	–	–	–	++			
Lam	Rabbit laminin	–	–	–	+			

The immunofluorescence reaction is scored subjectively from negative (–) to strongly positive (+++).
*Human keratin polypeptide numbers used as assigned by Moil *et al.*
†Positive on only 2% to 5% of cultured cells.

normal human urothelial turnover is estimated to occur at a rate of once every year, one of the lowest turnover rates of mammalian epithelia.[25] The potential for urothelial cell proliferation has been well documented. Wong and Martin, in a model of bladder injury, showed that mitotic activity occurs within 24 hours in the basal layer of the epithelium adjacent to the wound site.[26] At the injury margin, the epithelium forms a rolled edge, from which a two-layered sheet of flat cells grows over the edematous injury site. Healing is effected within about 1 week, as mitotic activity declines. Confirmatory studies with scanning electron microscopy showed that new epithelium spreads from a rolled epithelial edge.[26] Sutherland *et al.*, in a model of bladder regeneration following transplantation of an acellular matrix, also showed that the urothelium from the native bladder grows across the acellular matrix surface, completely relining the matrix patch within 4 days.[27]

What is the mechanism behind this urothelial proliferation? We have developed a model of bladder injury in the rat, surgically cutting the anterior bladder in half followed by primary repair (Fig. 15.1).[28] Using RNase protection assay, we measured the relative amounts of the message for keratocytic growth factor (KGF), showing that at 24 hours after injury KGF is elevated eight times more than control levels (Fig. 15.2).[28] Interestingly, in our model the posterior nonwounded bladder halves also showed an increase in KGF/mRNA expression, but to a lesser degree (six times higher than control levels). This

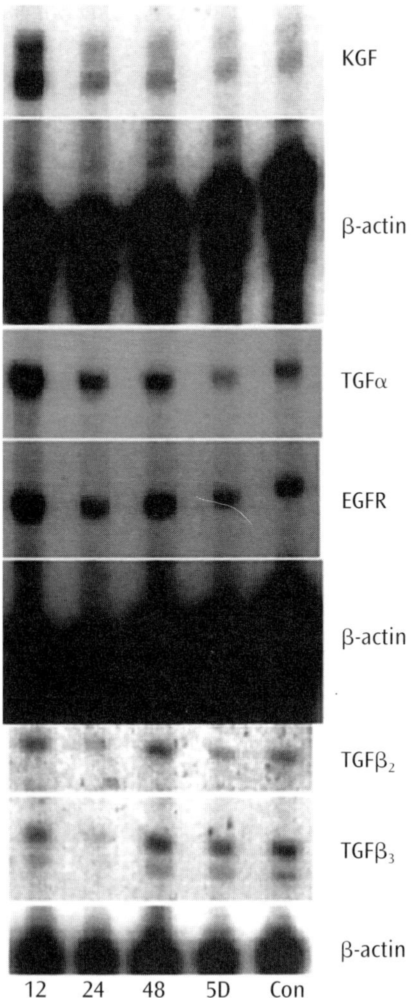

Figure 15.2 *Growth factor RNase protection assay in bladder wound healing. Note the increase in mRNA at 12 hours for KGF and TGFα. 12, 24, 48 represent hours, and 5D = 5 days after bladder injury. Con = control. Reproduced with permission from Baskin, L.* et al *(1997) Growth factors in bladder wound healing.* Journal of Urology, ***157****, 2388–95.*

implies that injury to the bladder evokes a response throughout the bladder wall, not localized exclusively to the immediate site of injury. In other words, bladder injury puts the entire urothelial population 'on guard.'

By 5 days after injury, the transcript levels for KGF had returned to baseline (i.e., the same as unoperated animals) in both the anterior wounded and posterior nonwounded bladder halves. This is consistent with the histologic data, in that urothelial proliferation and coverage of the urothelial defect are complete by 4 days in this bladder injury model. Transcripts for KGF receptor did not change as a function of injury. TGFα also was elevated early on in bladder wound healing, whereas $TGF\beta_2$ and $TGF\beta_3$ mRNA were not regulated as a function of bladder injury. Thus, the TGFβ isoforms do not appear to have a role during bladder wound healing.

These results are consistent with previously published data on growth factors in the bladder, as well as on changes in growth factor expression in the skin.[29,30] Werner *et al.* showed an approximately 100-fold increase in mRNA encoding KGF 1 day after surgical skin injury.[29] Furthermore, the increase in the KGF message was unique, in that the other members of the fibroblast growth factor family (FGF), acidic FGF (FGF-1), basic FGF (FGF-2), and FGF-5, were only slightly elevated during wound healing, and FGF-3, FGF-4, and FGF-6 were unchanged. In contrast to other FGF peptides, KGF acts in a strict paracrine fashion, with the receptor located on the epithelium and KGF secreted from the mesenchyme.[31,32] This is consistent with the stromal (fibroblast or smooth muscle) bladder cells producing the KGF, which in turn acts on the KGF receptor located in the urothelium, causing proliferation to repair the injury.[30]

STROMAL CELLS

Just as the phenotype of the urothelium can be defined, so can the stromal compartment. Previously, we have defined the ontogeny of smooth muscle development in the rat bladder.[33] Using immunohistochemical techniques, the expression of the smooth muscle proteins α actin, desmin, vinculin, vimentin, myosin, and laminin were defined as a function of development. As noted above, smooth muscle based on α actin localization is first noted at 16 days' gestation. The first mesenchymal marker to be detected in the rat bladder was vimentin at 15 days of gestation. With time, vimentin expression became localized exclusively to the fibroblasts of the lamina propria and connective tissue between the smooth muscle bundles. A similar pattern of expression has been reported in the developing stroma of the rat prostate and seminal vesicle, where vimentin is initially widely expressed in the mesenchyme, but, with time, localizes to the interductal connective tissue and lamina propria.[34]

Other investigators have also shown that smooth muscle cell differentiation, as defined by the temporal expression of smooth muscle markers, follows an orderly pattern. For example, McHugh and coworkers showed that there is a tissue-specific expression of the isoactin multigene family in the developing rat.[35] Specifically, they were able to show that both 'α' and 'γ' smooth muscle actin is first expressed at about 16 days gestation in the bladder of the fetal rat, consistent with our immunohistochemical studies.[33] In the rabbit bladder, Chiavegato *et al.* have shown that vimentin and an isoform of myosin are expressed in the embryonic period. However, with normal aging, these smooth muscle cell markers cease to be expressed but can reappear in the pathologic state of experimental obstruction.[36] Other smooth muscle markers, such as desmin, laminin, and vinculin, have also been shown to be developmentally and pathologically regulated.[37,38]

EXTRACELLULAR MATRIX

The extracellular matrix in the bladder also changes as a function of development and pathology. For example, collagen types I and III are the major interstitial collagens within the bladder wall. The amount and ratio of these structural collagens are regulated during development and in the poorly compliant bladder.[39–41] Aging also affects the extracellular matrix, with specific changes in the ultrastructure of the submucosa.[42,43] Elastic fiber proteins such as elastin, fibrillin 15, and microfibril-associated glycoprotein are also regulated as a function of development and location.[44]

Adhesion molecules in the bladder wall also play an important role in the required distensibility of the urinary bladder.[45] The normal human urothelial cell and/or its plasma membrane contains the integrins a3, aV, b1, and b4, but do not contain the integrin b3. The urothelial basement membrane contains collagen type IV and laminin. Fibronectin and the integrins a3 and b4 are found in or near the urothelial basement membrane area, with types I and III collagen and tenascin abutting the area. The patterns of collagen, laminin, tenascin, vitronectin, fibronectin, and the a3, aV, b1, and b3 integrins in the lamina propria, vessels, nerves, and smooth-muscle layers of the bladder may facilitate the cellular interactions that occur between the urothelial and stromal cells.

MESENCHYMAL–EPITHELIAL INTERACTIONS

We believe that bladder augmentation with intestine leads to abnormal cellular interactions between the urothelium and the foreign stroma. Over time, the phenotype of the urothelium will change and, in the worst case, lead to dysplasia or even cancer. We are now in the process of testing this hypothesis experimentally. Currently, however, there exists a large body of scientific evidence to support this concept. For example, when embryonic or, even more surprisingly, adult bladder epithelium is placed in direct contact with urogenital sinus mesenchyme, the bladder epithelium is induced to differentiate into glandular epithelium that resembles prostatic epithelium histologically, and ultrastructurally expresses androgen receptors, and secretes prostate-specific proteins.[46–9]

Change in the extracellular matrix environment of the stroma can profoundly influence adult epithelial morphology and function. This possibility has been recently tested by transplanting neonatal rat seminal vesicle mesenchyme to the cut end of the mouse adult ureter.[50] The adult urothelium was induced to undergo seminal vesicle morphogenesis, to express seminal vesicle cytodifferentiation, and to produce the complete spectrum of major seminal vesicle proteins characteristic of the mouse. The induced seminal vesicle epithelium also expressed androgen receptors which are not seen in urothelial tissue. Staining with Hoechst dye 33258, which can distinguish cells of mouse and rat origin, further demonstrated that the induced seminal vesicle

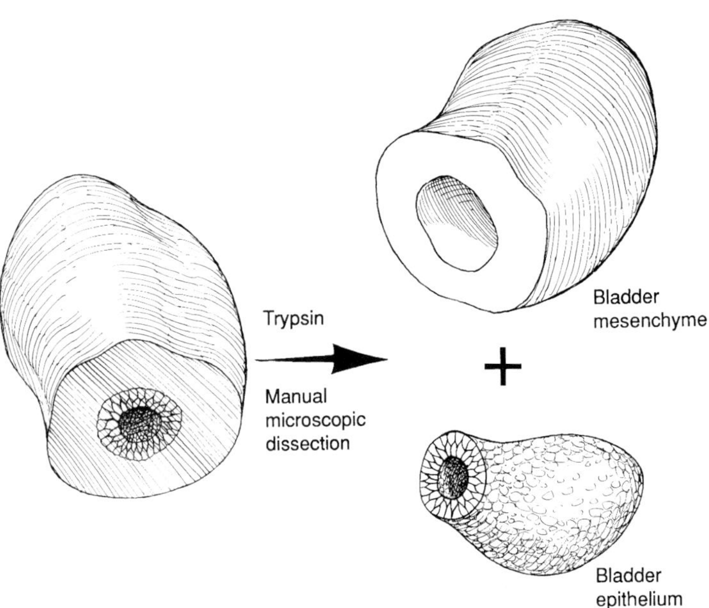

Figure 15.3 *Algorithm: tissue recombination experiments. 14-day gestation bladders were separated into bladder mesenchyme and the bladder urothelium by enzymatic tryptic digestion and manual separation of the urothelium from the mesenchyme by microscopic dissection. Reproduced with permission from Baskin, L.* et al *(1996) Role of mesenchymal–epithelial interactions in bladder development.* Journal of Urology, ***156****, 1820–7.*

epithelium was indeed of mouse origin and not a contaminant of the inducing rat seminal vesicle mesenchyme. In addition, neonatal mouse vaginal mesenchyme was grafted *in situ* beneath the bladder mucosa of adult male mice. The vaginal mesenchyme implanted into the bladders induced prostate-like acini, indicating that the above reprogramming of adult organs *in situ* is not an isolated occurrence. Similarly, a prostate-inducing mesenchyme has been compartmentalized into the fibromuscular wall of the urinary bladder, resulting in the induction of prostatic epithelium. We believe that the reciprocal communication between the epithelium and the stroma can lead to changes in the phenotype of each compartment, with the final outcome of inappropriate signaling being carcinogenesis.[51,52]

Adult mammary epithelium is also responsive to its stromal environment.[53] Normally, mammary epithelium differentiates into an alveolar branching ductal system with the epithelial cells secreting milk protein. In a series of tissue recombination experiments between mammary epithelium and various heterotypic embryonic mesenchymes (preputial glans, foot skin, tail skin, genital tubercle skin, mammary gland) and neonatal mesenchymes (uterus, vagina, and urinary bladder), Cunha *et al.* have shown that mammary growth and branching morphogenesis are altered to variable extents by different mesenchymes.[53] Furthermore, the ability to form alveoli and produce milk proteins in adult mammary epithelial cells is critically dependent upon the nature of the connective tissue environment.[53]

Not only is the mesenchyme critical for determining the epithelial phenotype, but the reciprocal interaction occurs with the epithelium determining mesenchymal differentiation. For example, we have shown that epithelium is necessary for the differentiation of bladder mesenchyme into bladder smooth muscle.[23] This was accomplished by growing 14–day embryonic bladder mesenchyme, with or without bladder epithelium, using previously described tissue separation and recombination techniques (Figs. 15.3 and 15.4).[23,54] Based upon immunocytochemical analysis of smooth muscle differentiation markers, these experiments showed that smooth muscle in the rat bladder was induced by the bladder epithelium.[33] Myometrial development is also dependent on the epithelium as an inducer via cell–cell interactions.[55]

We hypothesize that epithelial–mesenchymal interactions during development continue as epithelial stromal interactions after birth. In numerous

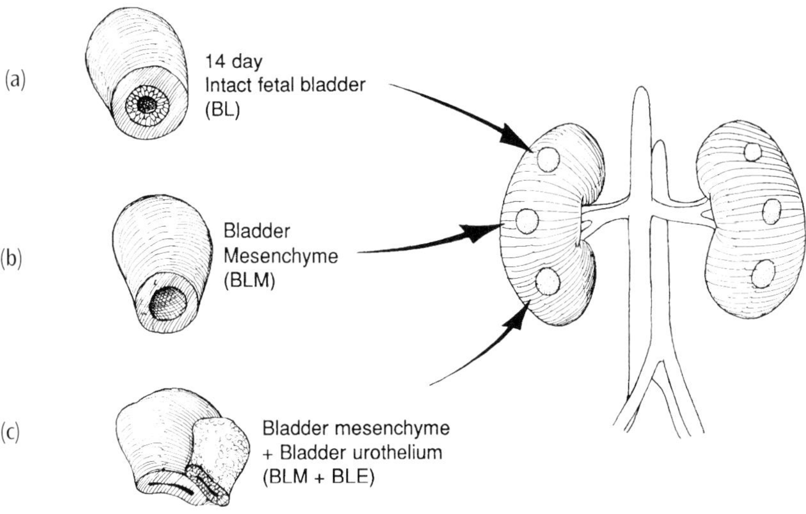

Figure 15.4 *Three types of tissue recombination specimens were prepared for grafting under the renal capsule of syngeneic hosts: (a) intact bladder (BL) which had been isolated from fetuses of timed pregnant rats (14 days' gestation) by surgical methods alone; (b) bladder mesenchyme (BLM) itself (urothelium removed following trypsinization and mechanical separation); and (c) isolated bladder mesenchyme recombined with bladder urothelium (BLM+BLE). Tissue recombinants (c) were prepared by transfering sheets of isolated bladder urothelium directly to the bladder mesenchyme and allowing the tissue layers to adhere during overnight culture on a solidified agar medium. Reproduced with permission from Baskin, L.* et al *(1996) Role of mesenchymal–epithelial interactions in bladder development.* Journal of Urology, ***156****, 1820–7.*

experimental systems, we know that the stroma regulates the epithelium, and the interactions are likely to be reciprocal.[56] For example, it has been suggested that both normal prostatic development and prostate carcinogenesis are mediated by stromal–epithelial interactions.[51,52] Recent evidence supporting this model comes from experiments in which the stroma surrounding prostatic tumors was analyzed by immunohistochemistry and shown to be dedifferentiated when compared to normal prostatic stroma.[57] In another experiment, Dunning tumor cells were placed in contact with different stromal environments. Compared to the nonstromal environment, there was a reduction in growth rate of the Dunning tumor cells and a loss of tumorigenesis demonstrated by both light microscopy and electron microscopy.[58] These findings demonstrate that the connective tissue environment can have profound regulative effects on neoplastic epithelial cells.

In the urinary bladder, it is likely that stromal–epithelial interactions play a role in tumorgenesis following augmentation enterocystoplasty. These tumors are primarily adenocarcinomas that originate on the bladder side of the anastomosis.[10] It is known that nitrosamines are elevated in the urine of patients who have undergone enterocystoplasty.[59] The nitrosamines, in turn, can cause mutagenic changes to the DNA. This hypothesis is supported by the increased incidence of cancer at the anastomotic site of patients who have had ureterosigmoidostomies.[60]

We propose an alternative hypothesis, that abnormal stromal–epithelial interactions at the site of anastomosis lead to perturbations in reciprocal cell-cell signaling between the intestinal stroma and the urothelium. *In vitro* studies on bladder cancer cell lines support this hypothesis. Gordon *et al.* showed that altered extracellular matrices influence human bladder cancer cell lines, possibly through regulation of the nuclear matrix.[61] The authors conclude that the extracellular matrices derived from transformed stroma-producing cells may influ-

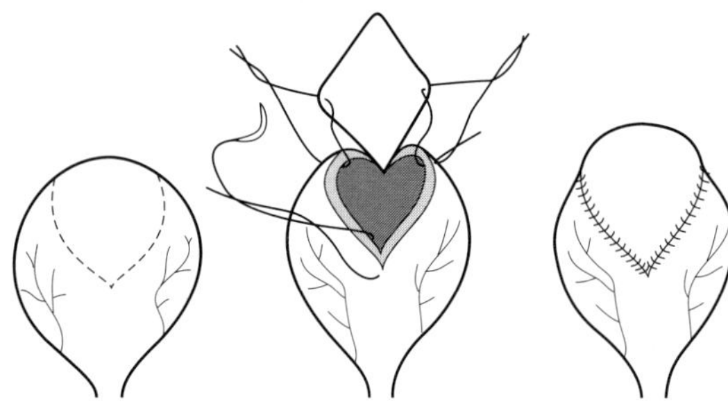

Figure 15.5 *Diagram of augmentation cystoplasty with acellular tissue matrix. Reproduced with permission from Sutherland, R.S.* et al *(1996) Regeneration of bladder urothelium, smooth muscle, blood vessels and nerves into an acellular tissue matrix.* Journal of Urology, ***156***, *571–7.*

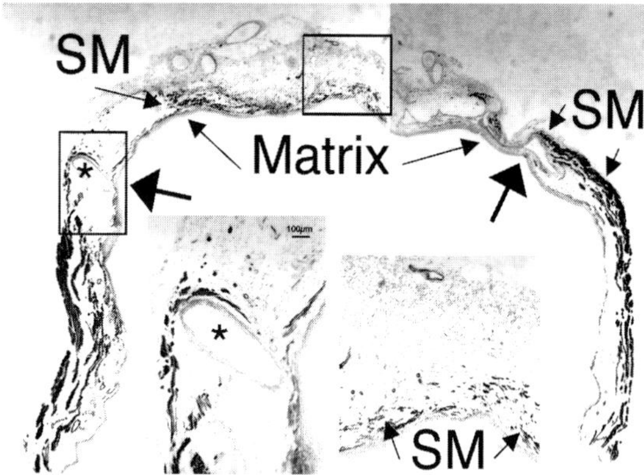

Figure 15.6 *Immunohistochemical localization (α-smooth muscle actin) of newly forming smooth muscle (SM) within the matrix 18 days after acellular matrix bladder augmentation. Note that urothelium has completely lined the acellular matrix. (* = suture sinus; small arrows denote new smooth muscle growth; and large arrows denote the native bladder acellular matrix junction. Reproduced with permission from Sutherland, R.S.* et al *(1996) Regeneration of bladder urothelium, smooth muscle, blood vessels and nerves into an acellular tissue matrix.* Journal of Urology, ***156***, *571–7.*

ence the proliferation, genetic regulation, and maintenance of the overlying urothelial tumor cells.

FUTURE DIRECTION

Regeneration of bladder tissue via an acellular tissue matrix

Clearly, a better solution to bladder augmentation needs to be found. We have developed a model of bladder wall regeneration using an acellular tissue matrix. This model consists of replacing the dome of the rat bladder with an acellular tissue matrix and analyzing the regeneration of bladder cells (smooth muscle, urothelium, vessels, and nerves) within this extracellular matrix scaffold (Fig. 15.5).[27] The acellular matrix tissue graft (~1 cm^3) is derived as a full-thickness segment from syngeneic rat gastric or bladder specimens. The acellular tissue matrix is prepared by removing the cellular elements with distilled water and mild detergent. The absence of stromal and epithelial cellular elements was confirmed histologically. A different type of acellular tissue matrix was developed by Badylak *et al.*, who used acellular porcine small intestinal submucosa (SIS).[62] While significant differences exist between SIS and the extracellular matrix scaffold that we have developed, both types of matrix grafts have been incorporated successfully into the bladder, becoming populated by both smooth muscle and urothelial cells. Thus, acellular tissue matrices derived from mammalian intestine or bladder can provide an excellent scaffold which facilitates cellular regeneration of the bladder.

In this model, extracellular matrix appears to organize the regenerative capacity of host bladder cells after bladder augmentation. The assumption in this model is that an appropriate extracellular matrix environment will allow urothelial cells from the native bladder to migrate into, and line, the acellular matrix patch. In turn, under the influence of the urothelium, stromal cells (smooth muscle or fibroblasts) from the native bladder invade and populate the acellular matrix. Along with the cellular infiltrates composed of urothelium, fibroblasts, and smooth muscle, a new vasculature develops that supplies nutrients to the regenerating bladder tissue.

Epithelialization of the acellular tissue matrix occurred by 4 days, accompanied by granulocytic infiltration (Fig. 15.6).[27] Smooth muscle regenerated within 2 weeks postgrafting when in juxtaposition to an epithelial surface, and matured into normal-sized bundles by 26 weeks. Neovascularity was seen by 2 weeks postsurgery. Neural elements formed around developing smooth muscle bundles as early as 4 weeks. The source of regenerative smooth muscle cells is most likely to be the host detrusor or muscularis mucosa, as witnessed by the apparent continuity with host tissues. It appears that existing host smooth muscle cells proliferate in response to local stimuli, and migrate into the adjacent graft. It is plausible that existing host smooth muscle cells undergo partial phenotypic dedifferentiation to a more primitive form, such as the myofibroblast, and then migrate. The spatial orientation of regenerating cellular elements suggests the presence of stromal–epithelial interactions taking place during phenotypic regeneration of the bladder. The fact that the smooth muscle is first noted adjacent to the urothelium supports the hypothesis that the urothelium plays a regulatory role in the formation of smooth muscle. This *in vivo* model provides a suitable means for the continued study of the stromal–epithelial interactions occurring during bladder cell regeneration.

REFERENCES

1. Wein, A.J., Levin, R.M. and Barrett, D.M. (1991) Voiding function and dysfunction. In Gillenwater, J. (ed.) *Adult and Pediatric Urology*, 2nd edn, Vol. 1. St Louis, Mosby: 933–1100.
2. Sutherland, R.S., Mevorach, A.R., Baskin, L.S. and Kogan, B.A. (1995) Spinal dysraphism in children: an overview and an approach to prevent complications. *Urology*, **46**, 294–304.
3. Baskin, L.S., Kogan, B.A. and Benard, F. (1990) Treatment of infants with neurogenic bladder dysfunction using anticholinergic drugs and intermittent catheterization. *British Journal of Urology*, **66**, 532–4.
4. Hinman, F.J. (1988) Selection of intestinal segments for bladder substitution: physical and physiological characteristics. *Journal of Urology*, **139**, 519–23.
5. Koch, M.O., McDougal, W.S., Hall, M.C. *et al.* (1992) Long-term metabolic effects of urinary diversion: a comparison of myelomeningocele patients managed by clean intermittent catheterization and urinary diversion. *Journal of Urology*, **147**, 1343–7.
6. Mundy, A.R. and Nurse D.E. (1992) Calcium balance, growth and skeletal mineralization in patients with cystoplasties. *British Journal of Urology*, **69**, 257–9.
7. Gosalbez, R.J., Woodard, J.R., Broecker, B.H. and Warshaw, B. (1993) Metabolic complications of the use of stomach for urinary reconstruction. *Journal of Urology*, **150** (2 Pt 2), 710–12.
8. Bogaert, G.A., Mevorach, R.A., Kim, J. and Kogan, B.A. (1995) The physiology of gastrocystoplasty: once a stomach, always a stomach. *Journal of Urology*, **153**, 1977–80.
9. Buson, H., Diaz, D.C., Manivel, J.C. *et al.* (1993) The development of tumors in experimental gastroenterocystoplasty. *Journal of Urology*, **150** (2 Pt 2), 730–3.
10. Barrington, J., Fulford, S., Griffiths, D. and Stephenson, T. (1997) Tumors in bladder remnant after augmentation enterocystoplasty. *Journal of Urology*, **157**, 482–6.
11. Blyth, B., Ewalt, D.H., Duckett, J.W. and Snyder, H. (1992) Lithogenic properties of enterocystoplasty. *Journal of Urology*, **148** (2 Pt 2), 575–7; discussion 578–9.
12. Cartwright, P.C. and Snow, B.W. (1989) Bladder autoaugmentation: partial detrusor excision to augment the bladder without use of bowel. *Journal of Urology*, **142**, 1050–3.
13. Buson, H.J., Manivel, J.C., Dayanc, M., Long, R. and Gonzalez, R. (1994) Seromuscular colocystoplasty lined with urothelium: experimental study. *Urology*, **44**, 743–8.
14. Nguyen, D.H., Mitchell, M.E., Horowitz, M., Bagli, D.J. and Carr, M.C. (1996) Demucosalised augmentation gastrocystoplasty with bladder autoaugmentation in pediatric patients. *Journal of Urology*, **156**, 206–9.
15. Baskin, L., Meaney, D., Landsman, A., Zderic, S. and Macarak, E. (1994) Bladder compliance increases with normal fetal development. *Journal of Urology*, **152**, 692–5.
16. Wu, X.R., Lin, J.H., Walz, T. *et al.* (1994) Mammalian uroplakins. A group of highly conserved urothelial differentiation-related

membrane proteins. *Journal of Biology, Chemistry,* **269**, 13716–24.

17. Baskin, L., Howard, P.S., *et al.* (1993) Effect of physical forces on bladder smooth muscle and urothelium. *Journal of Urology,* **150** (2 Pt 2), 601–7.
18. Hutton, K.A., Trejdosiewicz, L.K., Thomas, D.F. and Southgate, J. (1993) Urothelial tissue culture for bladder reconstruction: an experimental study. *Journal of Urology,* **150**, (2 Pt 2), 721–5.
19. de Boer, W.I., Schuller, A.G., Vermey, M. and vn der Kwast, T.H. (1994) Expression of growth factors and receptors during specific phases in regenerating urothelium after acute injury in vivo. *American Journal of Pathology,* **145**, 1199–207.
20. Southgate, J., Hutton, K.A., Thomas, D.F. and Trejdosiewicz, L.K. (1994) Normal human urothelial cells in vitro: proliferation and induction of stratification. *Laboratory Investigations,* **71**, 583–94.
21. Fujiyama, C., Masaki, Z. and Sugihara, H. (1995) Reconstruction of the urinary bladder mucosa in three-dimensional collagen gel culture: fibroblast–extracellular matrix interactions on the differentiation of transitional epithelial cells. *Journal of Urology,* **153**, 2060–7.
22. Southgate, J., Kennedy, W., Hutton, K.A. and Trejdosiewicz, L.K. (1995) Expression and in vitro regulation of integrins by normal human urothelial cells. *Cellular Adhesion and Communications*, **3**, 231–42.
23. Baskin, L.S., Hayward, S., *et al.* (1996) Role of mesenchymal–epithelial interactions in bladder development. *Journal of Urology,* **156**, 1820–7.
24. Hicks, R.M. (1975) The mammalian urinary bladder: an accommodating organ. *Biological Review, Cambridge Philosophical Society* **50**, 215–46.
25. Hainau, B. and Dombernowsky, P. (1974) Histology and cell proliferation in human bladder tumors. An autoradiographic study. *Cancer*, **33**, 115–26.
26. Wong, Y.C. and Martin, B.F. (1977) A study of light and scanning electron microscopy of the lining epithelium of the guinea pig bladder following artificial ulceration. *American Journal of Anatomy,* **150**, 219–35.
27. Sutherland, R.S., Baskin, L.B., Hayward, S.W. and Cunha, G.R. (1996) Regeneration of bladder urothelium, smooth muscle, blood vessels and nerves into an acellular tissue matrix. *Journal of Urology*, **156**, 571–7.
28. Baskin, L., Sutherland, R., Thomson, A. *et al.* (1997) Growth factors in bladder wound healing. *Journal of Urology,* **157**, 2388–95.
29. Werner, S., Smola, H., Liao, X. *et al.* (1994) The function of KGF in morphogenesis of epithelium and reepithelialization of wounds. *Science*, **266**, 819–22.
30. Baskin, L.S., Sutherland, R.S., Thomson, A. *et al.* (1996) Growth factors and receptors in bladder development and obstruction. *Laboratory Investigation*, **75**, 157–66.
31. Rubin, J.S., Osada, H., Finch, P.W. *et al.* (1989) Purification and characterization of a newly identified growth factor specific for epithelial cells. *Proceedings of the National Academy of Science, USA,* **86**, 802–6.
32. Finch, P.W., Cunha, G.R., Rubin, J.S., Wong, J. and Ron, D. (1995) Pattern of keratinocyte growth factor and keratinocyte growth factor receptor expression during mouse fetal development suggests a role in mediating morphogenetic mesenchymal–epithelial interactions. *Developmental Dynamics*, **203**, 223–40.
33. Baskin, L.S., Hayward, S.W., Young, P. and Cunha, G.R. (1996) Ontogeny of the rat bladder: smooth muscle and epithelial differentiation. *Acta Anatomica*, **155**, 163–71.
34. Hayward, S.W., Baskin, L.B., Haughney, P.C. *et al.* (1996) Stromal development in the ventral prostate, anterior prostate and seminal vesicle of the rat. *Acta Anatomica,* **155**, 94–103.
35. McHugh, K.M., Crawford, K. and Lessard, J.L. (1991) A comprehensive analysis of the developmental and tissue-specific expression of the isoactin multigene family in the rat. *Developing Biology,* **148**, 442–58.
36. Chiavegato, A., Scatena, M., Roelofs, M. *et al.* (1993) Cytoskeletal and cytocontractile protein composition of smooth muscle cells in developing and obstructed rabbit bladder. *Experimental Cell Research,* **207**, 310–20.
37. Allen, K.M. and Haworth, S.G. (1989) Cytoskeletal features of immature pulmonary vascular smooth muscle cells: the influence of pulmonary hypertension on normal development. *Journal of Pathology,* **158,** 311–17.

38. Glukhova, M., Koteliansky, V., Fondacci, C., Marotte, F. and Rappaport, L. (1993) Laminin variants and integrin laminin receptors in developing and adult human smooth muscle. *Developing Biology,* **157**, 437–47.
39. Ewalt, D.H., Howard, P.S., Blyth, B. *et al.* (1992) Is lamina propria matrix responsible for normal bladder compliance? *Journal of Urology,* **148** (2 Pt 2), 544–9.
40. Baskin, L.S., Constantinescu, S., Duckett, J.W., Snyder, H.M. and Macarak, E. (1994) Type III collagen decreases in normal fetal bovine bladder development. *Journal of Urology,* **152**, 688–91.
41. Howard, P.S., Ewalt, D.H.Duckett, J.W., Snyder, H.M. and Macarak, E.J. (1995) Alterations in extracellular matrix gene expression in normal versus non-compliant human bladders. *Advances in Experimental and Medical Biology*, **385**, 215–22; discussion 223–8.
42. Levy, B.J. and Wight, T.N. (1990) Structural changes in the aging submucosa: new morphologic criteria for the evaluation of the unstable human bladder. *Journal of Urology,* **144**, 1044–55.
43. Levy, B.J. and Wight T.N. (1995) The role of proteoglycans in bladder structure and function. *Advances in Experimental Medical Biology*, **385**, 191–205.
44. Rosenbloom, J., Koo, H., Howard, P.S., Mecham, R. and Macarak, E.J. (1995) Elastic fibers and their role in bladder extracellular matrix. *Advances in Experimental Medical Biology*, **385**, 161–72.
45. Wilson, C.B., Leopard, J., Cheresh, D.A. and Nakamura, R.M. (1996) Extracellular matrix and integrin composition of the normal bladder wall. *World Journal of Urology,* **14**, S30–7.
46. Donjacour, A.A. and Cunha G.R. (1988) Seminal vesicle mesenchyme induces prostatic morphology and secretion in urinary bladder epithelium. *Journal of Cell Biology,* **107**, 609a.
47. Donjacour, A.A. and Cunha, G.R. (1993) Assessment of prostatic protein secretion in tissue recombinants made of urogenital sinus mesenchyme and urothelium from normal or androgen-insensitive mice. *Endocrinology*, **131**, 2342–50.
48. Cunha, G.R., Sekkingstad, M. and Meloy, B.A. (1983) Heterospecific induction of prostatic development in tissue recombinants prepared with mouse, rat, rabbit and human tissues. *Differentiation*, **24**, 174–80.
49. Neubauer, B.L., Chung, L.W., McCormick, K.A. *et al.* (1983) Epithelial–mesenchymal interactions in prostatic development. II. Biochemical observations of prostatic induction by urogenital sinus mesenchyme in epithelium of the adult rodent urinary bladder. *Journal of Cellular Biology*, **96**, 1671–6.
50. Lipschutz, J., Young, P., Taguchi, O. and Cunha, G. (1996) Urothelial transformation into functional glandular tissue in situ. *Kidney International*, **49**, 59–66.
51. Cunha, G.R., Hayward, S.W., Dahiya, R. and Foster, B.A. (1996) Smooth muscle–epithelial interactions in normal and neoplastic prostatic development. *Acta Anatomica*, **155**, 63–72.
52. Hayward, S.W., Cunha, G.R. and Dahiya, R. (1996) Normal development and carcinogenesis of the prostate: a unifying hypothesis. *Annals of the New York Academy of Sciences,* **784**, 50–62.
53. Cunha, G.R., Young, P., Hamamoto, S., Guzman, R. and Nandi, S. (1992) Developmental response of adult mammary epithelial cells to various fetal and neonatal mesenchymes. *Epithelial Cell Biology*, **1**, 105–18.
54. Cunha, G.R. and Donjacour, A.A. (1987) Mesenchymal–epithelial interactions: technical considerations. In Coffey, D.S., Bruchovsky, N., Gardner, W.A., Resnick, M.I. and Karn, J.P. (eds). *Assessment of Current Concepts and Approaches to the Study of Prostate Cancer*. New York, A.R.Liss: 273–82.
55. Cunha, G.R., Young, P. and Brody, J.R. (1989) Role of uterine epithelium in the development of myometrial smooth muscle cells. *Biolology Reproduction*, **40**, 861–71.
56. Cunha, G.R., Bigsby, R.M., Cooke, P.S. and Sugimura, Y. (1985) Stromal–epithelial interactions in adult organs. *Cell Differentiation,* **17**, 137–48.
57. Hayward, S.W., Olumi, A.F., Haughney, P.C., Dahiya, R. and Cunha, G.R. (1996) Prostate adenocarcinoma causes dedifferentiation of its surrounding smooth muscle. *Proceedings of the American Urological Association,* **155**, 605A.
58. Cunha, G.R., Hayashi, N. and Wong, Y.C. (1991) Regulation of differentiation and growth of normal adult and neoplastic epithelia by inductive mesenchyme. *Cancer Survey*, **11**, 73–90.

59. Nurse, D.E. and Mundy, A.R. (1989) Assessment of the malignant potential of cystoplasty. *British Journal of Urology,* **64**, 489–92.
60. Crissey, M.M., Steele, G.D. and Gittes, R.F. (1980) Rat model for carcinogenesis in uretero-sigmoidostomy. *Science,* **207**, 1079–80.
61. Gordon, J.N., Shu, W.P., Schlussel, R.N., Droller, M.J. and Liu, B.C. (1993) Altered extracellular matrices influence cellular processes and nuclear matrix organizations of overlying human bladder urothelial cells. *Cancer Research*, **53**, 4971–7.
62. Badylak, S., Lantz, G., Coffey, A. and Geddes, L. (1989) Small intestinal submucosa as a large diameter vascular graft in the dog. *Journal of Surgical Research,* **47,** 74–80.

Index

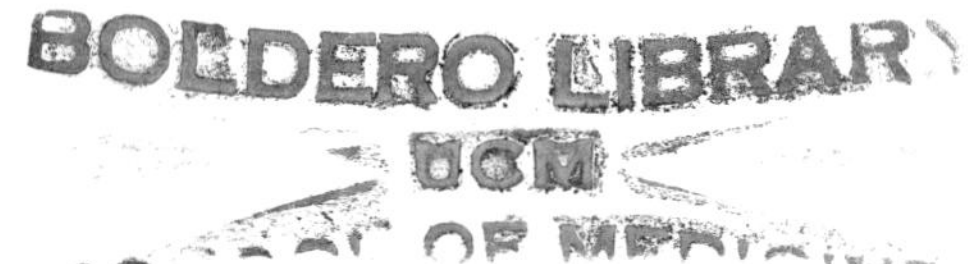